Super Fitness for Sports, Conditioning, and Health

Thomas D. Fahey, Ed.D.
California State University, Chico

Allyn and Bacon
Boston ■ London ■ Toronto ■ Sydney ■ Tokyo ■ Singapore

This book is dedicated to the memory of my parents.
They were always there for me when I needed them.

Vice President and Editor-in-Chief: *Paul A. Smith*
Publisher: *Joseph E. Burns*
Series Editorial Assistant: *Sue Walther Jones*
Marketing Manager: *Rick Muhr*
Production Editor: *Christopher H. Rawlings*
Editorial-Production Service: *Omegatype Typography, Inc.*
Composition and Prepress Buyer: *Linda Cox*
Manufacturing Buyer: *Dave Repetto*
Cover Administrator: *Jenny Hart*
Electronic Composition: *Omegatype Typography, Inc.*

Library of Congress Cataloging-in-Publication Data
Fahey, Thomas D. (Thomas Davin)
   Super fitness for sports, conditioning, and health / Thomas D. Fahey.
      p. cm.
   Includes bibliographical references and index.
   ISBN 0-205-31354-X (pbk.)
   1. Physical fitness. 2. Exercise. 3. Health. I. Title.
GV481.F275 2000
613.7′1—dc21   99-047647
                                       CIP

Printed in the United States of America

10 9 8 7 6 5 4 3 2 1   04 03 02 01 00 99

CONTENTS

3   Developing Endurance   26

4 Developing Muscle Strength 39

5 Developing Power and Speed 60

PREFACE

Super Fitness for Sports, Conditioning, and Health was written for those who want more from their exercise programs. A growing number of people are not satisfied with the couch potato lifestyle; they want to be active. They enjoy a variety of sports activities, such as dancing, cycling, hiking, skiing, playing volleyball, rollerblading, and golfing. Furthermore, they want to be good at them. If you follow the advice in this book, you will be able to run faster, jump higher, and perform better in the activities you love. And you can achieve these goals with surprisingly little effort.

Over the past 50 years, sports scientists, coaches, and athletes have developed an array of training techniques to improve strength, power, speed, endurance, flexibility, and skill. During the Cold War, scientists in Eastern bloc and Western countries competed as they developed almost superhuman Olympic athletes who could run faster, jump higher, and throw farther. Their research produced the following training techniques: plyometrics, downhill running, parachute sprinting, interval training, Olympic lifting, overdistance training, medicine ball training, motor unit overload techniques, PNF stretching, and exotic forms of resistive exercise training. These training methods are presented to you in this easy-to-read, comprehensive book.

Before you begin your training program, you need to learn how your body functions during exercise. The first two chapters of *Super Fitness* present an overview of basic exercise physiology and new information concerning exercise and health. In these chapters, you will learn how to get the most from your body when you spike a volleyball, lay up a basketball, sprint, or run a marathon. *Super Fitness* presents principles of exercise training that will make your program more fun and will help you achieve the body and fitness you want.

The chapter on endurance fitness will show you how to measure your fitness using simple techniques you can do in your neighborhood park, swimming pool, or running track. The interval and overdistance training techniques presented here will allow you to go faster and longer when you play your favorite sports. Training methods, which can be applied to any endurance sport, are described for running, swimming, and cycling.

The strength training chapter teaches you basic techniques for developing strength that can be done in as little as 20 minutes. Research has shown that, with these techniques, you can build all the strength you need in a fraction of the time it takes in traditional programs.

Chapters 5 and 6 are the most revolutionary sections of the book. They reveal techniques that, until a few years ago, Soviet scientists and coaches used secretly. For many years, most coaches did not have good techniques for improving sprint speed, quickness, or jumping ability. Yet Eastern European scientists and coaches had developed neuromuscular overload techniques that improved speed, quickness, and explosiveness and, consequently, had incredible success in Olympic sports. Now, these techniques are available to you. Practicing these simple exercises will help you move faster on the tennis court, hit a golf ball farther, and ride your mountain bike faster up a hill. If you work hard enough, you might even be able to slam dunk a basketball like Michael Jordan. The techniques are simple, fun, and effective.

The chapter on flexibility presents the science and techniques behind effective stretching exercises. You will learn how your body becomes more flexible, and you will read about the best exercises for rapidly achieving good joint flexibility.

Super Fitness gives you plenty of options for your program—more options than you could possibly include in a single exercise program. The chapter on program design gives suggestions for combining exercises that help you meet your sports and fitness goals.

The final chapter of *Super Fitness* gives you the straight scoop on sports nutrition and supplements. Sports scientists have developed some effective nutritional techniques that will help fuel your body for better performance. In addition to these nutritional techniques, you will get the latest information on popular supplements such as creatine monohydrate, androstenedione, and amino acids. This chapter also presents the risks and benefits of drugs, such as anabolic steroids, growth hormone, insulin, and IGF-1, used by athletes. You will learn basic dietary strategies that will enhance your health while providing energy for sports and daily activities.

Why listen to me? I have been involved in sports and exercise as a sports scientist, athlete, and coach for over 40 years. I am a coauthor of several leading college textbooks on exercise physiology, fitness and wellness, and weight training. As a sports scientist, I have traveled to Eastern European countries, such as Russia and Poland, many times to study their revolutionary techniques. As an athlete, I competed in track-and-field and weight lifting in college and continue to compete in Masters track-and-field today. I am currently the Master's U.S. National and Nike World Games champion and single-age American record-holder in the discus throw. I am also a university-level track-and-field coach. In short, I have a unique blend of theoretical and practical experience that can help you get the most from your training program.

The Surgeon General has said that exercise is the most important lifestyle habit you can have to improve your health. Using the techniques in this book, you can enhance your health and improve your performance at the same time, so get fit and have fun!

Acknowledgments

A book is always the product of not only the author's hard work but also the contributions of numerous other individuals. I would like to thank the production staff at Allyn and Bacon for their hard work on this project. I would also like to thank the following reviewers: Sally Dellinger, Ohio State University; Vicki Highstreet, University of Nebraska–Lincoln; Jeffery Hogan, University of California–Davis; Meg Lanchantin, University of North Carolina; John Linderman, Ohio State University–Columbus; Brian Pritschet, Eastern Illinois University; Richard Schroeder, De Anza College; Frank Verducci, San Francisco State University; and Carl Wallin, Dartmouth College. I would like to thank Monica Galvis for shooting most of the photographs. I am deeply indebted to the professors who have guided me in my education. They include Franklin Henry, G. L. Rarick, Frank Verducci, Vic Rowen, Allen Abraham, Bill Harkness, and especially George Brooks. George has been my friend and inspiration and fully deserves the Olympic prize in sports medicine. My coaches have a special place in my heart for the time and energy they devoted to my athletic and personal development. They include Bob Lualhati, Carl Wallin, Larry Burleson, Dick Trimmer, Bob Johnson, Tom Carey, and Arner Gustafson. I also want to recognize some of the many athletes with whom I have competed and coached. I have learned more about sports from them on the playing field than I have in a laboratory setting. These athletes include John Powell, Art Burns, Rich Schroeder, Dave MacKenzie, Bob Fritz, Brian Oldfield, Jack Kaserian, Mac Wilkins, Carl Wallin, John McDonald, Scott O'Brien, Dick Hodgkiss, Chad Morgan, Tim Fua, Chandra Flinn, Carley Pridham, Larry Kennedy, Jim McGoldrick, and Richard Marks. I especially want to remember two great athletes who passed away recently—Matt Goss and Joe Keshmiri. Both achieved great success in athletics, were fierce competitors, and died before their time.

Super Fitness

Many people are hooked on fitness. They run, ride bicycles, play tennis, and ski. Although some people work out to improve fitness for sports, others exercise simply to enhance their appearance. Even people who are inactive often want to start a training program. Whether you are currently inactive or an exercise fanatic, physical fitness will help you live an active lifestyle and enhance your health.

Physical fitness, the capacity to increase metabolism and meet the demands of physical effort, largely determines your quality of life. Fitness gives you freedom—freedom to move your body the way you want. Physically fit people have more energy, are less susceptible to many diseases, and can better enjoy many sports, such as skiing, hiking, or cycling.

Even if you do not like sports, you need physical energy and stamina to work, tour a museum, or stay up late studying for an exam. Physically fit people have stronger bones as they age, have less back trouble, can perform daily tasks more effectively, and are more mentally alert. Regular exercise can dramatically reduce the risk of many diseases and health problems related to aging.

Fitness is essential to metabolic health. Your body is basically a self-contained chemical factory. Chemical reactions help process fuels, build and break down tissues, and enable communication among different parts of the body. The physically fit person's body can better manage these chemical processes. Efficient management of body chemistry prevents diseases, such as atherosclerosis and diabetes (non-insulin-dependent diabetes), improves your ability to manage body fat, and prevents deterioration of muscle and bone mass as you age.

Fitness in the Age of the Couch Potato

When it comes to fitness, Americans have a split personality. Many people often avoid exercise, blaming their busy schedules and competing activities, such as using computers or watching television, for their inactivity. These people develop an inactive lifestyle as they spend hours on the Internet or watching their favorite television shows. Studies show that totally inactive people would benefit greatly from even a light exercise program.

On the other hand, for many people exercise is an important part of their lives. They work out regularly, play sports, maintain a healthy weight, do not use tobacco products, and eat a well-balanced diet. This fitness subculture is highly visible in its quest for toned, healthy-looking bodies. Across the United States and Canada, people belong to comprehensive health clubs that offer weight training, aerobics, swimming, basketball, and racquetball. These fitness enthusiasts flock to tennis courts, golf courses, and ski resorts; they participate in a variety of activities and sports. In addition, they strive to develop good health and healthy-looking bodies. Fitness is central to their lives.

This book is for people who want to develop physical fitness, but it does not neglect the novice. If you are a beginner, you will learn basic principles for incorporating exercise into your life. You will learn no-nonsense techniques for developing a basic level of physical fitness without having to train for hours in a strenuous exercise program, techniques that highlight the advantages of becoming more physically active during the course of your daily activities. As you will see, you can attain the benefits of improved fitness with surprisingly little effort.

Good health is a goal of almost everyone. In addition to good health, most people who exercise regularly want healthy-looking bodies and improved physical fitness for activities they enjoy, such as skiing, volleyball, basketball, hiking, and swimming; these people are not content with a basic level of fitness. They play a variety of sports and need greater fitness to help them in their activities. They want a leaner, healthier look and realize that exercise is essential to attaining this goal.

Whether your goal is to develop fitness for health or performance, this book is for you. You will learn the most up-to-date methods of achieving a high level of fitness so that you look and feel better, and you will be able to enhance your performance in your favorite sports or recreational activities. During the past 30 years, advances in sports medicine have improved athletic performance to spectacular levels. Using these techniques, you can rapidly and safely improve fitness for health and performance.

Surgeon General's Report on Fitness

It is official; the U.S. Surgeon General has determined that lack of exercise is hazardous to your health. In 1996, the U.S. government issued "The Surgeon General's Report on Physical Activity and Health,"[1] a landmark document stating that regular, moderate activity can dramatically reduce the risk of many diseases and health problems.

Regular exercise may be the single most important lifestyle activity for attaining a healthier, more disease-resistant body. The Centers for Disease Control

---

[1]U.S. Department of Health and Human Services. *Physical Activity and Health: A Report of the Surgeon General.* Atlanta, GA: U.S. Department of Health and Human Services, Centers for Disease Control and Prevention, National Center for Chronic Disease Prevention and Health Promotion, 1996.

TABLE 1.1 **Some Major Health Benefits of Regular Exercise**

Reduced risk of premature death (all causes)
Reduced risk of coronary heart disease
Influences on other risk factors of coronary heart disease
- Reduces blood pressure
- Lowers body fat
- Lowers blood fats
- Increases HDL (protective substance)
- Reduces platelet stickiness (platelets are a blood component)
- Reduces effects of stress
- Improves glucose tolerance (related to a type of diabetes)
- Encourages healthy living habits
Reduced risk of some types of cancer
Improved mental health
Prevented or delayed osteoporosis
Prevented or improved symptoms of arthritis
Prevented muscle and nerve deterioration with aging

and the Surgeon General stated that regular exercise is perhaps the single most important lifestyle practice you can do to enhance wellness. Table 1.1 summarizes ways that regular exercise may enhance health.

Exercise lowers the risk of premature death. People who exercise experience a lower death rate from all causes, including the leading killers—coronary heart disease and cancer—and accidents.

Exercise reduces the risk of developing coronary heart disease. People who exercise have a lower risk of developing and dying from heart disease. Active people also have a lower risk of developing hypertension (high blood pressure), an important risk factor for heart disease and stroke. Regular exercise affects the risk factors for heart disease; physical activity lowers cholesterol and low-density lipoproteins ("bad" cholesterol), raises high-density lipoproteins ("good" cholesterol), reduces the risk of developing non-insulin-dependent diabetes (problems with sugar metabolism), makes blood platelets (blood components important in forming blood clots) less sticky, and helps reduce body fat. Exercise also reduces the risk of heart disease for people who smoke cigarettes.

Exercise reduces the risk of developing some types of cancer. Physical activity during work or leisure lowers the risk of developing colon cancer. Researchers claim that exercise affects this type of cancer by speeding up the transit time of food through the gastrointestinal tract. Several studies have shown a possible link between physical activity and a reduced risk of breast cancer and perhaps other reproductive cancers. Physical activity during high school and college years may be particularly important for preventing breast cancer during adulthood.

However, too much physical activity can also be problematic. Some types of cancer may be related to problems with the immune system, your body's mechanism for fighting disease. Doing too much exercise on a chronic basis, a condition sometimes called *overtraining*, may impair your immune system and increase your risk of developing some types of cancer. Unfortunately, scientists know little about the effects of overexercise on disease.

Regular exercise improves mental health.   Exercise helps relieve symptoms of depression and anxiety and improves mood and sense of well-being. Increasingly, mental health professionals use exercise as an inexpensive way to treat patients.

Exercise may prevent osteoporosis and increase or maintain muscle mass during aging.   Osteoporosis is characterized by loss of bone mass. Exercise during growth and early adulthood helps increase or maintain bone mass, which may be important in preventing postmenopausal bone loss.

In older people, exercise helps preserve muscle mass and movement skills, which can prevent accidents and life-threatening fractures. If you are inactive, by age 70 you can expect to lose 20 percent of your active muscle tissue. The connection of nerve and muscle is lost in many motor units. Fast-twitch motor units, necessary for powerful movement, gradually switch to less powerful slow-twitch motor units. Strength training can prevent much of this deterioration that occurs with age.

Exercise may prevent arthritis and help people who have the disease.   Physical activity is important for maintaining joint mobility in people who have osteo- and rheumatoid arthritis. If the program is not too severe, exercise can reduce symptoms of these diseases. Exercise helps to maintain the health of tissues lining the joints and facilitates joint lubrication.

Surgeon General's Exercise Recommendations

The Surgeon General's report recommended that "People of all ages should do at least 30 minutes of physical activity of moderate intensity (such as brisk walking) on most, if not all days of the week." The report also stated, "Greater health benefits can be obtained by engaging in physical activity of more vigorous intensity or of longer duration." Furthermore, "Cardiorespiratory endurance activity (such as walking, running, or swimming) should be supplemented with strength-development exercises at least twice per week for adults, in order to improve musculoskeletal health, maintain independence in performing the activities of daily life, and reduce the risk of falling."

The basic findings and recommendations in the Surgeon General's report should not be news. Most of us realize that exercise is good for our health and that we should do it regularly. Nevertheless, only 15 percent of people do regular, vigorous exercise. Over 60 percent of adults are not regularly physically active, and 25 percent do not exercise at all. Half of young people ages 12 to 21 do not exercise vigorously on a regular basis. Among high school students, participation in daily

physical education classes decreased from 42 percent in 1991 to 25 perce
The problem is most severe among young women and gets worse for both
throughout the teenage years. By college, young men and women approach t
ercise levels of the adult population (U.S. Department of Health and Human
vices, 1996).

Healthy People 2000

In 1990, the federal government issued its health goals for the turn of the century
entitled "Healthy People 2000." This report set the following three major goals: increase the span of healthy life for U.S. citizens, reduce health disparities among U.S.
citizens, and achieve access to preventive services for all U.S. citizens. Two additional recommendations were to increase the activity level of the average U.S. citi-
zen and to increase the proportion of people who exercise vigorously.

Developing Physical Fitness

Developing aerobic capacity has been the primary goal of recreational exercisers
since Kenneth Cooper published his landmark book *Aerobics* in 1965. This book,
based on hundreds of studies conducted since the early 1900s, defined fitness as
the body's ability to transport and use oxygen. Aerobic capacity is also known as
cardiorespiratory capacity. The quest for aerobic fitness led to popular exercise crazes,
such as jogging, beginning in the 1970s, and aerobics classes, beginning in the 1980s.
Aerobic capacity, however, is only one dimension of fitness.

Today, fitness experts realize that it is not quite that simple. In addition to aerobic capacity, other components of fitness are vital to health and performance.
These include muscle strength and power, muscle endurance, flexibility, and body
composition.

The Fitness Components

Aerobic or Cardiorespiratory Capacity

The ability to supply energy for activities lasting more than 30 seconds depends on
the consumption and use of oxygen (O_2). Most physical activities in daily life and
athletics take more than 90 seconds, so O_2 consumption is critical for survival as
well as performance. Oxygen consumption increases as we go from rest to light exercise to intense exercise. The maximum rate that you consume O_2, called *maximal
oxygen consumption* or $\dot{V}O_{2max}$ (a symbol meaning the volume of oxygen consumed
per minute), is one of the most important factors determining how vigorously you
can exercise, how long you can sustain exercise, and how fast you recover.

Aerobic capacity includes two components—*oxygen transport capacity* and *cellular endurance capacity.* Oxygen transport capacity is the ability to move oxygen
from the air to the cells. It depends on well-functioning lungs, heart, and blood

ır endurance capacity is the ability of the cells to consume oxygen,
nd generate energy for cell functions, such as muscular work (see

durance capacity is an important part of aerobic capacity because
y supply energy for exercise. Oxygen consumption and much of
production occur in the cells' mitochondria. Mitochondria allow
to consume oxygen and use fat as fuel; they also protect your cells against destructive chemicals called *free radicals*, which may cause aging.

EXERCISING TO DEVELOP AEROBIC CAPACITY.   Endurance exercise best develops both components of aerobic capacity. Examples include walking, running, swimming, cycling, and cross-country skiing. Sports activities such as tennis, volleyball, soccer, and basketball also develop aerobic capacity.

High-intensity endurance exercise develops oxygen transport capacity most effectively. A general recommendation for developing oxygen transport capacity includes:

- *Mode of activity.*   Do aerobic exercise, such as running, cycling, swimming, or cross-country skiing.
- *Frequency of training.*   Exercise 3 to 5 days per week.
- *Intensity of training.*   Train at 55/65–90 percent of maximum heart rate, or 40/50–85 percent of maximum oxygen uptake reserve. The lower-intensity values (55–64 percent of maximum heart rate and 40–49 percent of maximum oxygen uptake reserve) are most applicable to people who are not physically fit or active. Athletes or people who desire extremely high levels of aerobic fitness often practice interval training at maximum intensity. Interval training involves repeated bouts of exercise at a relatively high intensity with brief rest periods between bouts.
- *Duration of training.*   Do 15 to 60 minutes of continuous aerobic activity. Duration is dependent on the intensity of the activity.

Overdistance training (prolonged endurance exercise) is best for developing cellular endurance capacity. People serious about developing high levels of cellular endurance will often run, cycle, or swim many miles in the quest for superior levels of endurance. Chapter 3 discusses the development of aerobic capacity and endurance in more detail.

Muscular Strength and Power

A second major component of fitness is *muscular strength*, or the ability to exert force. Closely related to muscular strength, *power* is the ability to exert force rapidly. In certain situations, power is more important than strength in helping people meet the physical requirements of daily life. For example, if an older person started to slip in the bathtub, his or her power capacity would be much more important than strength in preventing the fall. The person would have to react quickly to prevent a serious fall or injury. Power is also important for people interested in participating in sports. For example, skiers, tennis players, and golfers must exert force rapidly to achieve maximum performance.

Another component, *speed*, is considered an important aspect of fitness. Speed, the ability to move rapidly, is actually the same thing as power. Fast movements, such as swinging a golf club or baseball bat, require you to exert as much force as possible at high speeds. The faster you move, the less force you can apply during the movement. However, the force is maximum for that speed. The speed of powerful movements depends on the load, or the resistance to movement.

Strength contributes significantly to wellness. It keeps your skeleton in proper alignment, helps you exert force and move more easily, and helps you maintain lean-body mass (fat-free weight).

Proper skeletal alignment is important for preventing back and knee problems. For example, if you have weak abdominal and back muscles, your pelvis tends to tilt forward more than usual, which puts pressure on sensitive spinal nerves and causes back pain. Weak quadriceps muscles (the muscles on the front of the thigh) can cause the kneecap to shift to the outside of the knee joint, a movement that causes pain to the undersurface of the bone.

Good muscle strength is essential for smooth, efficient performance of everyday activities. Carrying groceries, lifting boxes, and walking up a flight of stairs are much easier if you have good muscle strength. In recreational activities, stronger people can hit the ball harder in tennis, get over an edge better in skiing, and jump higher in volleyball.

Good muscle strength helps maintain a higher lean-body mass (fat-free weight), an important component for the control of body composition. Scientists have discovered that the rate we use energy relates to lean-body mass, which consists mainly of muscle. Increasing muscle mass through strength training will make it easier for you to keep body fat low and under control.

STRENGTH AND AGING. After age 30, people start to lose muscle mass. At first, you notice that you cannot play sports as well as you could in high school. With years of inactivity and loss of strength, you may even have trouble performing simple movements required in everyday life. Some people eventually have trouble getting out of a tub or automobile, walking up a flight of stairs, or working in the yard. With poor strength, it is easy to slip in the tub or hurt your back when lifting objects.

As you age, motor nerves (the nerves that activate muscle fibers) become disconnected from individual muscle fibers. Muscle physiologists estimate that, for most people, by age 70, 15 percent of the motor nerves become disconnected from their muscle fibers. Doing strength exercises can prevent much of this loss.

Your muscles have fast and slow motor units. Quick, powerful movements require large, fast motor units; slower movements, such as maintaining posture, use smaller, slower motor units. In older muscles, the slower motor units start to take over, making powerful movements more difficult. Doing strength exercises prevents muscles from becoming slower due to inactivity.

Practicing resistance exercise, whether you use weights, weight machines, or your own body weight as resistance, is important for fitness and wellness. Strength training makes your movements more powerful, helps maintain muscle mass (important for weight control), and contributes to healthy joints.

STRENGTH AND WELLNESS.   Almost everyone should do some exercise to develop the major muscle groups and maintain good joint health. People should do strength exercises at least two times a week. Even doing simple resistance exercises that require no equipment, such as knee bends and push-ups, will help to insure good muscle and joint health.

STRENGTH AND PERFORMANCE.   People who want to improve sports performance will often benefit from resistance exercise programs that develop muscles important in their sport. However, improving sports performance is mainly a matter of improving skill. Increased strength is valuable in sports only if it can be incorporated with increased skill.

Muscular Power

Power has long been a neglected component of fitness even though it is critical for good performance in most sports. You will be amazed at how fast your performance and general movement skills improve if you concentrate on power. In endurance sports, you will be able to run, swim, and bike faster. In other sports, you can hit a golf or tennis ball harder, jump higher, and move quicker when you have more power. Many factors affect power, including strength, muscle size, muscle elasticity, skill, and body mechanics.

MUSCULAR POWER AND WELLNESS.   Accidents are a leading cause of death at any age. To avoid these problems, rapid, powerful movements are often required. Everyday actions, such as recovering your balance when you slip on a wet surface, are impossible if you do not have adequate muscular power. Good power also makes movements easier, which helps maintain your energy level during the day.

MUSCULAR POWER AND PERFORMANCE.   Muscular power is critical for performance in most sports. Simply practicing the sport is the best way to improve sports-specific power. Serious athletes benefit from exercises that force the muscles to exert force rapidly.

EXERCISING TO DEVELOP POWER.   For people interested in fitness for health and wellness, doing general strength exercises will improve muscular power adequately. People who want more power for sports and better movement should do specialized power exercises. These exercises will be presented in detail in Chapters 3, 5, and 6. Examples of power exercises include:

- *Plyometric exercises.*   During these exercises, you repeatedly and suddenly load your muscles and then immediately contract them. Examples include repeated standing long jumps, hops, vertical jumps, and box jumps.

■ *Speed exercises.*   These exercises force you to exercise at maximum power output. They overload the muscles you use during maximum effort. Examples include the high knee sprint exercise (vigorously lift your knees while driving your arms in a sprinting motion), bounding sprint strides with vigorous hip extensions, rope skipping, and downhill sprinting (sprinting down a 2–3 percent grade).

■ *Interval training.*   During these exercises, you perform repeated bouts of sprints for short distances, ranging from 20 yards to 1 mile. In an interval training program, you might run eight 440-yard dashes in 80 seconds with 5 minutes of rest between runs.

Muscular Endurance

Muscular endurance is the ability to sustain a given level of muscle force. This ability is important for tasks such as standing or sitting for long periods. It depends on a combination of muscle strength and cellular endurance capacity. Muscle endurance is best developed by frequently repeating an exercise and practicing sports and activities requiring a lot of muscle endurance.

MUSCULAR ENDURANCE AND WELLNESS.   Good muscular endurance is important for preventing low back and neck pain. Fit muscles can help maintain the spine in a position that prevents pressure on sensitive spinal nerves and maintains good health of the spinal joints. You develop adequate muscle endurance when you faithfully practice endurance and strength exercises.

MUSCULAR ENDURANCE AND PERFORMANCE.   In sports, muscular endurance is important in activities requiring sustained muscle contractions, such as snow and water skiing, wrestling, and rock climbing. As with muscle power, muscular endurance is best developed by practicing the sport or movement. However, you can build this fitness component by doing many repetitions of exercises that develop muscles used in the activity.

Flexibility

Flexibility is the ability to move joints through their ranges of motion. Flexibility is important for joint health, and this component helps maintain the normal range of motion of the major joints of the body.

FLEXIBILITY AND WELLNESS.   Flexibility helps maintain joints and muscles in their proper alignment, which may prevent common back disorders and joint deterioration due to aging. Maintaining normal range of motion also promotes joint lubrication, an essential factor in metabolism in joint soft tissues.

FLEXIBILITY AND PERFORMANCE.   Flexibility helps prevent injury and often improves movement capacity. For example, baseball pitchers with greater shoulder flexibility can exert force through a greater range of motion, and thus throw the ball harder. Many movements in gymnastics and dance are impossible without adequate flexibility. Flexibility for sports is developed best by practicing the specific movements, but you can also enhance flexibility by doing stretching exercises for the muscles and joints used in the activity.

Body Composition

The ideal body composition is one that has an acceptable level of body fat for your age and sex and a high proportion of lean-body mass. Lean-body mass is fat free and mainly composed of skeletal muscle. Skeletal muscle is not only essential for muscle strength but is also a high-energy tissue that helps keep body fat under control.

BODY COMPOSITION AND WELLNESS.   Excessive body fat can lead to many health problems, such as an increased risk of coronary heart disease, hypertension, stroke, joint problems, diabetes, gall bladder disease, cancer, injury proneness, and back pain. The American Heart Association has classified obesity as a leading risk factor for developing coronary artery disease.[2] Unfortunately, losing body fat is very difficult for most people.

Research studies have shown that the best way to lose weight and keep it off is to have a lifelong program of sensible diet and exercise. The diet should be low in fat, balanced, and contain enough calories to maintain a balance between energy input and energy output. The ideal exercise program should include endurance, strength, and flexibility exercises so that you burn calories, maintain a high metabolic rate, and remain free of injury.

BODY COMPOSITION AND PERFORMANCE.   The ideal body composition is different for each sport. For example, champion male and female distance runners typically have about 7 and 14 percent fat, respectively. Champion shot-putters of both genders often carry more than 20–25 percent fat. Body composition control for athletes uses the same principles as for anyone else—controlling food intake, energy expenditure, and muscle mass.

Which Fitness Component Should You Emphasize?

The structure of your exercise program depends on your fitness goals. If your goal is good health, your main goal should be to do some physical activity every day. Plan ways to become more active. For example, park several blocks away from

---

[2]The other leading risk factors for developing coronary artery disease include hypertension, physical inactivity, high blood fats (high cholesterol or triglycerides, low high-density lipoproteins), diabetes, and cigarette smoking.

work or school instead of parking in the lot next door. Take the stairs instead of the elevator. Mow the lawn yourself instead of hiring someone else to do it. Take some time every day for a walk or jog. Make physical activity a critical part of your life.

If you enjoy recreational activities, such as rock climbing, analyze the physical requirements of the sport and develop the appropriate type of fitness program. The rock climber needs muscle endurance, so doing high-repetition weight training exercises is appropriate. Rock climbers must be able to lift their own body weight; therefore, include pull-ups, push-ups, and squats. You also need endurance, so walking up hills or using a stair-climbing machine might be beneficial.

If you are a body builder or want to have a more attractive body, you probably want to have low body fat and toned muscles. Balance all the components of fitness. You need power to maximize muscle fitness as well as aerobic and cellular fitness to help you control your body composition and enhance your health.

If you are interested in strength–speed sports (e.g., tennis, basketball, volleyball, skiing), emphasize power and do not do too many overdistance exercises because this will cause you to lose speed. Do not neglect skill development, and structure your program so that you prevent athletic injuries before they occur.

Distance athletes (e.g., marathon runners) must develop cellular endurance capacity but cannot neglect the other fitness components. Successful endurance athletes have relatively low body fat, yet they need a lot of energy for activity. Therefore, you have to structure your diet very carefully.

Exercising only a small amount every day brings health benefits. Recent research has shown that if you are interested in fitness only for health, you can get considerable benefits by merely being more physically active during the day. Accumulating 30 minutes a day of almost any exercise can prevent heart disease and extend your life. This concept is discussed in Chapter 3.

No single fitness program is right for everyone. Some people want to do only enough exercise to look good. Others exercise to improve health. Still others want to develop high levels of strength or endurance for sports. Analyze your fitness goals; then systematically develop each of the fitness components you need for success. Almost everyone can benefit from an exercise program. You will get the most from your activity program if you plan ahead. This book will help you assess your fitness needs and teach you to develop an exercise program that produces the results you want.

Putting the Exercise Program in Its Proper Perspective

Many people work to develop the perfect body and high levels of fitness. The good news is that anyone can improve fitness with a well-structured exercise program. The bad news is that not everyone can have the body of a fashion model or bodybuilder or achieve Olympic levels of fitness. Genetic and motivational factors often limit people's abilities to achieve a lean, muscular body or superior strength, endurance, and power. Do the best you can, and do not expect perfection. The most important thing is to be physically active and enjoy the process. If you learn all you can about exercise training, you will make satisfactory progress toward developing a healthy, attractive-looking body and a higher level of physical fitness.

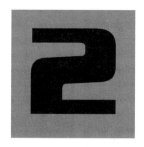

Exercise and Your Body

Your body is involved in a constant balancing act with its internal chemistry. It must balance the rate it builds and breaks down tissues, and it must provide enough energy for the many physical processes necessary to sustain life. It breaks down foods to supply energy, but it also stores energy in the liver, fat cells, and muscle for later use. Exercise, pumping blood, and breathing require energy. Energy helps destroy worn-out cells and tissues and builds new ones; it also regulates body water balance, sends nervous signals, and fuels thought processes. The total of all the chemical processes occurring in the body is called *metabolism.* Without energy from metabolism, you could not run, throw a ball, lift weights, or go for a walk.

Physical fitness is the capacity to increase metabolism and meet the demands of physical effort. Exercise increases your metabolic rate—the harder you exercise, the more it accelerates. At rest, you have a low metabolic rate, but it increases as you stand up and walk. When jogging, your metabolic rate increases more than 800 percent above your metabolic rate at rest. Olympic-caliber distance runners and cross-country skiers can increase metabolism by a startling 2,000 percent or more.

Physically fit people excel at metabolic management. They can rapidly supply energy for powerful movements and maintain healthy physical systems. Unfit people, on the other hand, cannot generate the energy needed for powerful or sustained exercise and are often subject to an array of physically deteriorating diseases. Their bodies cannot cope with substances produced during intense physical activity, so they tire easily. Consequently, their legs hurt, and they breathe heavily walking up a flight of stairs. Recreational activities, such as skiing or tennis, are difficult or impossible for them because they lack basic physical stamina.

Muscle power is also closely related to your capacity to increase metabolic rate. Power is the rate at which you can exert force. Muscle power depends on muscle size, the rate your nervous system can activate the muscles, muscle coordination, and the ability of chemical factors within the muscles to withstand fatigue.

Energy Management and Exercise

Machines work by converting one form of energy to another. The automobile engine, for example, works by transforming chemical energy (gasoline) into mechanical energy (the movement of the pistons). The human body works in a similar way. It takes chemical energy from food and converts it into other forms of energy useful to the body, such as mechanical work. These energy conversions might allow the body to contract muscles, conduct nerve impulses, or renew bone cells or muscle protein.

Food, such as a sandwich or chocolate bar, contains energy. Digesting the food and releasing all the energy would be wasteful because the body cannot use all of it at once. As a result, your body stores the energy in forms it can use more gradually. The most basic form of storage energy is *adenosine triphosphate* or *ATP*.

ATP is the *energy currency* of the cell—it supplies energy for the majority of the body's physiological processes. Rather than use the energy released from foods directly, the body traps energy as ATP. When the body needs energy for processes such as muscle contraction, the manufacture of new proteins, or the control of fluid levels in the cells, it breaks down ATP. ATP releases the energy that fuels biological processes, such as muscle contractions (Figure 2.1).

Foods are classified as fats, carbohydrates, and proteins. After a meal, you store excess energy that is not used to make ATP. *Fats* are stored in adipose tissue (fat cells). *Carbohydrates* help maintain blood sugar (*glucose*) and are stored as *glycogen,* an important energy supplier during exercise. This substance is stored mainly in the liver, skeletal muscle, and kidneys. *Amino acids,* the basic units in proteins, are not stored as fuel; rather, they are constructed into protein structures throughout the body. They can also be broken down for energy or incorporated into carbohydrate or fat energy stores.

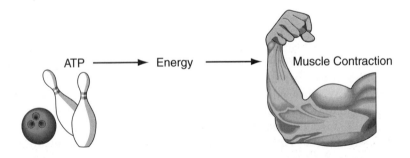

ATP ⟶ Energy ⟶ Muscle Contraction

FIGURE 2.1   Converting Energy from Storage.   Energy released from ATP breakdown fuels muscle contraction.

Fats, carbohydrates, and proteins can be broken down later to form new ATP to accommodate increases in metabolic rate. When you exercise, your need for ATP is great. Consequently, you mobilize your energy stores to increase ATP production.

Exercise and the Three Energy Systems

The body has three energy systems to carry out life processes: *immediate, nonoxidative,* and *oxidative.* These systems also perform specific functions during exercise. Your body uses the immediate energy system to exercise for three seconds or less; examples of exercises in this category include weight lifting, shot-putting, or discus throwing. The nonoxidative system, on the other hand, is used for speed events that last 3–60 seconds, such as the 100 and 400 meter runs. For events lasting longer than 2 minutes, such as distance running or swimming, the oxidative system is used.

Except for short power events, such as weight lifting, your body uses all three energy systems concurrently whenever you exercise. For example, when you play tennis, your body uses the immediate energy system when hitting the ball, but replenishes energy stores using the nonoxidative and oxidative systems.

The Immediate Energy System

The components of the immediate energy system include ATP and *creatine phosphate (CP).* During exercise, ATP breaks down and releases energy that is used to contract your muscles. You do not have much ATP, so the stores are replenished immediately by breaking down CP. During even the most intense exercise, ATP levels stay high, but CP levels deplete rapidly. After a few seconds, you reach the maximum capacity for this system and must use the nonoxidative and oxidative energy systems to restore ATP and CP levels. Switching to the other energy systems is essential because the muscles will stiffen (a condition called *rigor*) and become unusable if you run out of ATP.

The Nonoxidative Energy System

The nonoxidative energy system makes new ATP by breaking down blood sugar (glucose) and glycogen stored in the muscles, liver, and kidneys. Because this system does not require oxygen, it is sometimes called the *anaerobic system.* The capacity of this system is also limited, but it can generate a lot of ATP in a short time. This capability makes it the most important energy system for intense exercise.

Two problems are associated with the nonoxidative energy system: (1) carbohydrate stores are limited, and (2) rapid use of the system produces substances that cause fatigue. Your brain and nervous system rely on carbohydrates to function properly; low blood sugar causes dizziness, fatigue, and poor judgment. During intense, prolonged exercise, such as playing 3–4 sets of tennis for 3–4 hours, you deplete your carbohydrates rapidly, making it difficult to exercise.

Intense exercise increases the production of *lactic acid*. Although lactic acid is an important fuel in the body, it releases substances called *hydrogen ions* that are thought to interfere with metabolism and muscle contraction. During heavy exercise, such as sprinting, you produce a lot of lactic acid and hydrogen ions, so you fatigue rapidly. Fortunately, exercise training helps your body cope with high levels of hydrogen ions and lactic acid.

The Oxidative System (Also Called the Aerobic System)

Unlike the nonoxidative energy system, the oxidative system requires oxygen to generate ATP. Although it cannot produce energy for exercise as fast as the other energy systems, it can supply energy for a longer period of time. Consequently, for activities lasting more than a few minutes, the oxidative system becomes critically important.

For this energy system to work, the body must transport oxygen from the air to the cells (Figure 2.2). Oxygen is transported to the cells through the blood stream

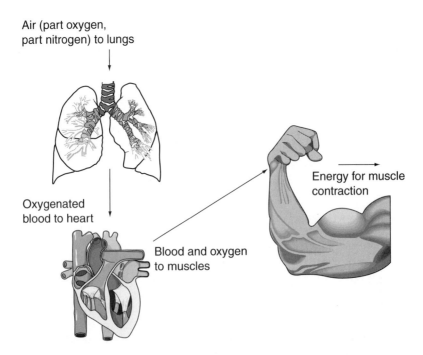

Air (part oxygen, part nitrogen) to lungs

Oxygenated blood to heart

Blood and oxygen to muscles

Energy for muscle contraction

FIGURE 2.2   The Transport of Oxygen.   Oxygen is transported from the air to the lungs and into the blood. The heart pumps oxygen-rich blood to the cells and then into the cell mitochondria. There, oxygen is used to help produce large amounts of ATP to fuel cellular processes.

by the cardiorespiratory system. This system requires healthy lungs to move the oxygen into the body and a strong, healthy heart to pump the oxygen-rich blood from the lungs to the cells. Exercise training increases the capacity of the heart to pump blood and, to a certain extent, increases the capacity of the lungs to move oxygen from the environment to the blood stream. When the oxygen reaches the cells, it is transported to cell structures called *mitochondria,* known as the power-houses of the cell because they produce most of its ATP. They contain enzymes that drive chemical reactions responsible for extracting energy from the foods we eat. The energy is captured in the form of ATP, and used for muscle contractions, the manufacture of new protein, and other cellular functions.

In a given sport, one of the energy systems will be most important. For example, weight lifters rely on the immediate energy system, sprinters depend on the nonoxidative system, and endurance runners predominantly use the oxidative system. Your exercise program should stress the energy system most important to your fitness goals.

Developing Metabolic Fitness

Metabolic fitness is the ability to provide energy to the muscles while exercising. For instance, if you want to improve your ability to run fast over short distances (i.e., sprint), you have to train your metabolism to supply a lot of energy in a short time. If your goal is to develop better endurance for hiking or backpacking, then you should train your metabolism to supply energy over a more sustained period of time. Training and the three energy systems are summarized in Table 2.1.

Physically fit people are good at generating ATP and managing metabolism, so they can exercise longer and more intensely. Exercise training causes the body to enhance many of the elements essential to ATP production.

When designing your program, consider your ultimate fitness goal. Exercises that develop oxygen metabolism tend to render health benefits. You would emphasize exercises that develop oxidative metabolism if you want to be a better hiker or

TABLE 2.1   The Three Energy Systems

	Power	Speed	Endurance
Duration of event	0–3 seconds	3 seconds–2 minutes	More than 2 minutes
Examples of event	Discus, shot put, weight lifting	100 to 400 meter run	1,500 meter run, marathon, triathlon
Speed of body chemistry	Immediate, very rapid	Rapid	Slower but prolonged
Types of fuel	ATP and CP	Muscle glycogen and glucose	Muscle and liver glycogen, glucose, fats, amino acids

distance runner. If you are interested in strength–speed sports, such as softball, throwing events, or soccer, then concentrate on the faster-energy systems.

Most people should do some exercise for each energy system. No sport or exercise relies completely on one system. The tennis player needs endurance to play for the entire match and the strength to hit powerful shots. The weight lifter must have strength to lift the weights and endurance to work-out for 1–2 hours. Likewise, distance swimmers need good endurance and must have enough speed and power to swim fast. Everyone, regardless of his or her favorite sport, needs some cardiovascular fitness for good health.

Developing Fitness for Power

Almost any motion fits into this category, which describes movements lasting less than 3 seconds. If you stand up from your chair, you use the immediate energy system to supply the energy for muscle contractions. Likewise, if you throw a softball as far as you can, you are using the immediate energy system. However, maximum effort lasting only a few seconds requires maximum activation of the immediate energy system. Training increases high-energy fuel stores, enhances the enzymes used to break them down, and improves the nervous system's ability to turn on the muscles. This type of fitness is particularly valuable for throwing events (i.e., discus, shot put, hammer, javelin), baseball or softball pitching, and weight lifting.

If you want to develop the capacity for powerful movement, do exercises that specifically overload this component. Even if the sport or exercise is repetitive, such as downhill skiing or tennis, you must have the muscle power to perform each movement. For example, to make 20 or 30 turns when skiing down a hill, you must have enough power to execute each turn.

You develop this immediate energy system fitness by doing exercises that develop high levels of muscle tension. Recent research suggests that merely having high levels of strength is not enough for powerful movements. You have to develop the capacity to exert force rapidly (Delecluse, 1997). Training for these activities might include weight training, plyometrics, short sprints (i.e., starts), or exercises that use your own body as resistance. These techniques are discussed in detail in Chapters 4–6.

Developing Fitness for Speed

The category *fitness for speed* includes sports and exercises lasting 3 seconds to 2 minutes. As discussed, these movements emphasize the nonoxidative energy system. You train the muscles to generate a lot of power for short bursts and to recover quickly. This type of fitness is valuable in tennis, football, basketball, volleyball, soccer, softball, field hockey, and downhill skiing. In these sports, the other energy systems are important as well and should also be trained.

Fitness for this metabolic component is best developed through interval training. *Interval training* involves repeated bouts of high-intensity exercises. Usually, a short rest occurs between each repetition of an exercise. Fitness is highly specific—overload your body the way you want it to adapt. Do cycling intervals if you want to improve fitness for cycling, and do swimming intervals if you want to swim faster. This type of fitness is also intensity specific. If your goal is to run faster for 800 meters, you will not improve much if you run repeated 800 meter trials at a slow pace or jog slowly for longer distances. If you want to move fast, train fast.

Developing Fitness for Endurance

To be considered an endurance exercise, motion must continue for more than 2 minutes. As you increase the duration of exercise, you begin to rely more on the oxidative energy system. This system requires lungs that can deliver oxygen to the blood stream, rid the body of carbon dioxide, and help control body-fatiguing hydrogen ion levels. You need a strong heart and blood vessels to transport blood rapidly to the cells, and you must have a well-developed chemical system within the cells to process fuels and oxygen rapidly.

Perhaps the most important benefit of endurance exercise is the improved ability of your heart, lungs, and circulatory system to carry oxygen to your body's tissues. Your heart pumps more blood per beat, blood volume increases, resting and submaximal exercise heart rate slows, the number of red blood cells increases, blood supply to the tissues improves, and resting blood pressure decreases. A fit cardiorespiratory system does not work as hard at rest and at low levels of exercise because it functions more efficiently. A trained heart can better withstand the stresses and strains of daily life and meet the occasional emergencies that make extraordinary demands on your body's cardiorespiratory resources.

The best measure of the body's capacity to deliver and use oxygen is *maximal oxygen consumption* ($\dot{V}O_{2max}$). $\dot{V}O_{2max}$ reflects your body's internal chemical capacity. Scientists measure $\dot{V}O_{2max}$ by how much oxygen a person extracts from the air during intense exercise on a treadmill or stationary bicycle.

Endurance training also develops cell mitochondria by increasing the size of this component of the cell. This helps you use more fat as fuel and consume more oxygen.

Although there is considerable overlap in training $\dot{V}O_{2max}$ and mitochondrial capacity, there are specific exercises that best promote each one. $\dot{V}O_{2max}$ is best developed through interval training. Generally, the length of the interval is 1–5 minutes of intense exercise. For example, a runner attempting to increase $\dot{V}O_{2max}$ might run 8 intervals of 400 meters at 90 percent of maximum capacity. A swimmer might swim 8 intervals of 100 meters at 90 percent. Depending on the fitness of the person, each interval might take 60–100 seconds.

Scientists have discovered that $\dot{V}O_{2max}$ depends on muscle power as well as the capacity of the heart and lungs to transport oxygen. Chemical processes within muscle that limit muscle power can cause fatigue and limit the ability of the heart and lungs to deliver oxygen to the tissues. Muscle power and oxygen transport capacity should be developed at the same time in order to exercise at high intensities during endurance exercise.

Mitochondrial capacity is best developed by overdistance training, sometimes known as *long-slow-distance training*. This training involves prolonged exercise lasting anywhere from 10 minutes to several hours. Again, overdistance training should be specific to the sport—runners should run, cyclists should cycle, and swimmers should swim.

Muscle Function during Exercise

The purpose of training the three energy systems is to increase muscle function and prevent fatigue during exercise. Muscles are connected by tendons. When a muscle contracts, it shortens and pulls on the tendon, making the bone move.

Muscles are made up of individual muscle cells connected in bundles. Muscle fibers are composed of subunits called *myofibrils* (Figure 2.3). The myofibrils are

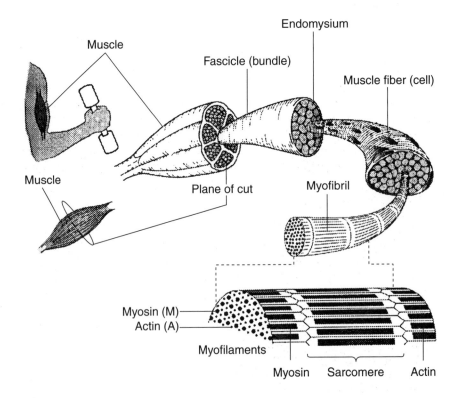

FIGURE 2.3   **Basic Muscle Structure.**

Adapted from Brooks, Fahey, White, and Baldwin (2000).

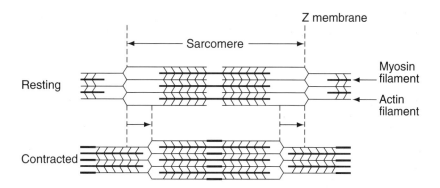

FIGURE 2.4   Muscle Contraction.   Muscles contract by shortening the sarcomeres, the basic contractile unit of the muscle fiber. Actin and myosin units slide past each other causing the muscle to shorten. The muscle pulls on the bones of the skeleton, causing movement.

divided into units called *myofilaments* (actin and myosin) that slide across each other to cause muscle contraction (Figure 2.4).

The Motor Unit

Nerve–muscle combinations called *motor units* generate muscle force and cause movement (Figure 2.5). Muscle fibers receive the signal to contract from nerves connected to the spinal column. To create the chain reaction in this network, a motor nerve (a nerve connected to muscle fibers) links as few as one or two muscle fibers or more than 150 muscle fibers. Powerful muscles, such as the quadriceps in the legs, have large motor units—each motor nerve connects to many muscle fibers. Smaller muscles, such as those found around the eye, have much smaller motor units.

The three types of motor units are fast glycolytic (FG), fast oxidative glycolytic (FOG), and slow oxidative (SO). They are subdivided according to their strength and speed of contraction, speed of nerve conduction, and resistance to fatigue. The type of motor unit chosen by the body depends on the requirements of the muscle contraction. For lifting heavy weights or sprinting, the body chooses FG fibers because they are fast and powerful. SO fibers, on the other hand, are chosen for prolonged standing or slow walking because they are more resistant to fatigue.

The body exerts force by signaling one or more motor units to contract, a process referred to as *motor unit recruitment.* When you want to pick up a small weight, for example, you use few motor units to do the task. However, when you want to pick up a large weight, you will use many motor units. When a motor unit calls upon its fibers to contract, all the fibers contract to their maximum capacity.

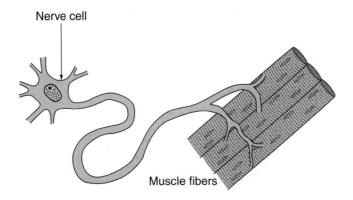

Nerve cell

Muscle fibers

FIGURE 2.5   The Motor Unit.

Increased Fitness through Improved Motor Unit Recruitment

Exercise training improves your nervous system's ability to coordinate the recruitment of muscle fibers. It is a kind of *muscle learning* and is an important way of increasing physical performance and skill. This form of exercise training increases muscle strength without greatly increasing muscle size. During the first weeks of weight training, most of the changes in strength are due to neurological adaptations, not increased muscle size.

Skilled performers in any sport or exercise execute movements by properly timing muscle contractions. In golf, for example, any person can hit the ball far by properly sequencing muscle movements. You can perform powerful movements when you can coordinate your muscle contractions at the proper time, when your muscles are strong and can be activated quickly, and when you have the metabolic fitness to complete the exercise.

Exercising only a small amount every day brings health benefits. Recent research has shown that if you are only interested in fitness for health reasons, you can get considerable benefits by merely being more physically active during the day. Accumulating 30 minutes a day of almost any exercise can prevent heart disease and extend your life. This concept is discussed in Chapter 3.

The Fitness Process: Exercise Training and Adaptation of the Body

Designing an exercise program for anyone requires a basic knowledge of the effects of exercise on the body. The basic principles of training for beginning exercisers and more experienced people are very similar. Both subject themselves to an exercise stress, and their bodies respond by increasing physical fitness. For example, the beginner's program might include a brisk walk or bicycle ride, whereas a serious athlete might bench-press 300 pounds or run 400 meters in 60 seconds. The process of stress and adaptation is the same for anyone who exercises, whether the person is a world-class athlete or a heart patient. Fitness improves by giving the body an unaccustomed exercise stress, such as walking instead of sitting, lifting a heavier weight, running faster or farther, or stretching a muscle more than usual. The body adapts to the stress by improving its function.

In the late 1940s, Dr. Hans Selye formulated the theory of stress adaptation, making a profound effect on medicine and having tremendous implications in conditioning for physical activity and sports. He called the process of stress adaptation the *general adaptation syndrome* (GAS). Selye described three processes involved in response to a stressor (something that upsets the body's balance, e.g., exercise, temperature, bacteria): alarm reaction, resistance development, and exhaustion.

The *alarm reaction* is the initial response to the stressor and involves the mobilization of the organism. During exercise, for example, your body reacts to the stress by breathing harder, sweating, and increasing the heart rate. The alarm reaction disturbs your physiology and disrupts your body's balance.

The *resistance development stage* is an attempt to adjust to the effects of the stressor. Your body improves its function so that the stressor is less disruptive to your physiology. For example, when you lift weights, your muscles get larger (hypertrophy) so that the load becomes less stressful. Resistance development is the goal of physical conditioning; you adapt only if the stress load disrupts your body balance. During exercise, if the stress is below a critical intensity, you do not improve your fitness. On the other hand, do not place too much stress on your body. If you cannot tolerate the training load, you become injured.

The amount and intensity of exercise necessary to improve fitness depend on fitness, age, health, mental outlook, and a number of unknown factors, such as genetics and blood hormone levels. For example, running a 10-minute mile may be exhausting to an inactive 40-year-old person, but this activity would cause essentially no adaptive response in a world-class distance runner. Likewise, a training run tolerated easily one day may be completely inappropriate on a day following a prolonged illness. Environment can also introduce intraindividual variability in performance. A person will typically experience decreased performance capabilities in extreme heat or cold, at high altitudes, or in polluted air.

If the stress is too great, then you enter the third stage of GAS, the *stage of exhaustion*. This stage is an excessive stress, either acute (applied all at once) or chronic (occurring over a period of time), that causes injury. Examples of acute exhaustion include fractures, sprains, and strains. Chronic exhaustion is more subtle and includes overtraining, stress fractures, and emotional stress.

Principles of Training

A number of factors influence how your body adapts to the stress of exercise. These include the degree of overload (how hard you push yourself), specificity of training

(training the way you want your body to adapt), individual differences (genetics), progression (taking it one step at a time), and reversibility (use it or lose it).

The Overload Principle

The basis of the general adaptation syndrome is that stressing the body to a tolerable limit causes adaptation and improved function. This positive stressor is an overload, quantified according to *load, repetition, rest,* and *frequency.* Load refers to the intensity of the exercise. Repetition refers to the number of times a load is administered. Rest refers to the time interval between repetitions. Frequency is the number of training sessions per week. For example, in weight training, you might do 3 sets of 8 different exercises using a weight you can barely lift for 10 repetitions (load and repetition), with 1 minute between each set (rest). You might do this workout 3 times per week (frequency). The nature of overload in an exercise program is not an exact science. Start conservatively and build up. The overload is excessive if you get injured, have trouble recovering, or are exceedingly sore.

Specificity of Training

The body adapts specifically to the stress of exercise. For example, the adaptation to endurance exercises, such as distance running or swimming, differs from that of strength exercises, such as weight lifting, and from power exercises, such as sprinting. Any training program should reflect the desired adaptation; train the way you want your body to change.

Doing the wrong type of training can actually impair certain types of fitness. For example, training for strength and endurance at the same time interferes with strength development. Although this is not a problem for a person exercising for improved health and appearance, it is an important consideration for a person trying to develop maximum strength and power.

Sports skills are extremely specific. Scientists have discovered that movement skills become ingrained in the nervous system and are *played back* by reflex. The aim of practice and coaching is to ingrain the correct motion; practicing incorrect motions develops the wrong patterns in your nervous system, resulting in incorrect movement patterns. The more a person practices a movement (up to a certain point on a learning curve, depending on the sport), the more it reinforces the skill in the nervous system. Therefore, it is imperative that you practice only correct movements (i.e., good technique).

Individual Differences

Anyone watching the Olympics, a professional football game, or a tennis match on the television can readily see that from a physical standpoint, we are not all created equal. Large individual differences in our ability to perform and learn sports skills become apparent. Genetics limits your capacity to develop fitness and skill. However, anyone can improve if he or she stays on a systematic program.

Genetics is also important for health and wellness. Some people are genetically more healthy than others; their immune systems naturally fight disease better than other people's. They are less susceptible to coronary heart disease, diabetes, and obesity, among other conditions. Even though you may be fortunate enough to have a family history of longevity and freedom from many diseases, lifestyle is far more important than genetics in determining health and well-being.

Progression

Adaptation to the stress of training occurs most readily when you apply the exercise stress gradually. High levels of fitness require many years of training and involve progression in small stages. Superior fitness and physical performance are the results of many small gains. You cannot become physically fit overnight, only gradually, one step at a time.

Reversibility

This principle is the reverse of the overload principle. Your body adapts to the stresses placed upon it. If you exercise more intensely than usual, then you improve fitness; if you do less, then you lose fitness. A graphic example of reversibility occurs when you wear a cast for a broken bone. When the doctor removes the cast, your arm or leg is much smaller than before because the muscles atrophy (get smaller) as a result of inactivity.

Develop Your Body to Suit Your Lifestyle

The human body is extremely adaptable. Determine what you want from an exercise program, and then mold your body in that direction. If your goal is health promotion and you do not want to begin a formal exercise program, structure your life so that you are more active during the day. If you have more lofty fitness goals, determine the elements that will help you achieve them.

Many people want to improve performance in recreational sports. If the sports you prefer require more endurance, concentrate on the oxidative energy system and endurance exercise. If you want to be a better tennis or volleyball player, you must not only develop skill but also work on muscle power and general endurance to improve your game. If you are mainly interested in improving your appearance, you must develop a healthy diet and exercise strategy to lose fat and maintain or gain lean-body mass. Exercise can be fun and rewarding, particularly if it helps you achieve your goals.

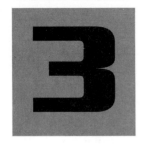

Developing Endurance

Endurance is an important fitness component for health and performance. If you do 30 minutes of endurance exercise a day, you will probably live longer, have a lower risk of heart disease and some types of cancer, prevent physical deterioration as you age, and improve your mental health.

You will most likely have more energy than inactive people to participate in a full day of activities. If you go to school, you will have the stamina to go to class, do your homework, and still have enough energy to enjoy yourself in your spare time. If you like to play tennis, volleyball, or basketball, you will have the ability to play your best with a lower risk of injury. When you are physically fit, you can go on a ski vacation, hit the slopes during the day, and go dancing at night without being exhausted. Endurance fitness allows you to play longer and harder and live a healthier, more vigorous life.

What Is Endurance Fitness?

Endurance is the capacity to sustain a given level of physical effort. Good endurance depends on the heart's and lungs' ability to deliver oxygen to the tissues (i.e., *aerobic capacity*) and the cells' ability to use oxygen and process fuels (i.e., *cellular endurance capacity*). Performance in endurance activities is also determined by *muscle power*. Good muscle power, combined with a strong heart and well-developed cell metabolic capacity, helps you exercise longer and faster.

Optimal development of the three components of endurance fitness (i.e., aerobic capacity, cellular endurance capacity, and muscle power) requires different training strategies. To increase aerobic capacity, do a combination of overdistance and interval training (discussed later in this chapter). To develop cellular endurance, do overdistance training. To improve muscle power, try interval training and resistance exercises. (Techniques for developing muscle power will be discussed in Chapters 4–6.)

Endurance Fitness and Maximal Oxygen Consumption

An important measure of endurance capacity is maximal oxygen consumption ($\dot{V}O_{2max}$); $\dot{V}O_{2max}$ measures your ability to deliver and use oxygen and your capacity to exercise at high intensities. Scientists measure $\dot{V}O_{2max}$ in sophisticated, exercise physiology laboratories using expensive treadmills, gas analyzers, and computers. During the test, you periodically increase the exercise intensity. Each minute, your oxygen intake, heart rate, breathing rate, and body temperature increase until you fatigue. Your highest level of oxygen consumption during the test is your maximal oxygen consumption.

During the test, the electrical activity of the heart is also measured (the electrocardiogram). This record helps your doctor determine if your heart is working correctly during exercise. Physicians will often perform an exercise electrocardiogram to assess the health of your heart or to determine if you can safely begin an exercise program.

Assessing Endurance Fitness

For most people, taking complicated, expensive exercise tests is not necessary. You can assess your endurance fitness using simple field tests, such as the 1 mile walking test, the Cooper 12 minute run, the 6 mile bicycle test, and the Cooper 12 minute swim test. Use these tests to assess your starting fitness and to measure progress in your program. Choose a test that reflects the nature of your exercise program; for example, if you plan to swim, take the swimming test rather than the running or walking test. You can estimate your fitness for walking, running, swimming, and biking with simple field tests. If you are starting an exercise program, take the walking test. If you have been exercising regularly, take one of the other field tests. Choose the test that most closely fits your favorite type of exercise. Once again, performance on the running field test will tell you little about your fitness for swimming.

You should see your physician before taking these tests if you:

- have heart trouble
- frequently suffer from chest pain
- have dizzy spells
- have high blood pressure
- have bone or joint problems
- are a male over 40 or a female over 50

1 Mile Walk Test

The 1 mile walk test is a good fitness test for a person beginning an exercise program (see Table 3.1). The best place to take this test is on a ¼ mile track (440 yards or 400 meters). If you do not have access to one, mark off a course on smooth, flat ground using your car odometer.

TABLE 3.1   1 Mile Walk Test

	Time (minutes: seconds)				
Males (yr.)	*High*	*Above Average*	*Average*	*Below Average*	*Low*
18–29	<13:00	13:00–16:00	16:01–18:45	18:46–22:00	>22:00
30–39	<13:00	13:00–16:00	16:01–19:00	19:01–22:00	>22
40–49	<13:30	13:31–16:15	16:16–19:15	19:16–22:15	>22:15
50–59	<14:00	14:01–16:45	16:46–19:45	19:46–22:45	>22:45
60–69	<14:30	14:31–17:15	17:16–20:15	20:16–23:15	>23:15
Females (yr.)	*High*	*Above Average*	*Average*	*Below Average*	*Low*
18–29	<13:30	13:30–16:30	16:31–19:15	19:16–22:30	>22:30
30–39	<13:30	13:30–16:30	16:31–19:15	19:16–22:30	>22:30
40–49	<14:00	14:01–16:45	16:46–19:45	19:46–22:45	>22:45
50–59	<14:30	14:31–17:15	17:16–20:15	20:16–23:15	>23:15
60–69	<15:00	15:01–17:45	17:46–20:45	20:46–23:45	>23:45

Source: Kline, G. M., J. P. Porcari, R. Hintermeister, P. S. Freedson, A. Ward, R. F. McCarron, J. Ross, and J. M. Rippe. 1987. Estimation of $\dot{V}O_{2max}$ from a one-mile track walk, gender, age, and body weight. *Med. Sci. Sports Exerc.* 19: 253–259.

Begin with some warm-up exercises, such as simple stretches and walking in place. Then, walk a mile as fast as you can. Using a stopwatch, time your walk to the nearest second. Because this is a walking test, you must always have one foot in contact with the ground. If both feet leave the ground at any time during the movement, you are running.

Cooper 12 Minute Run

The Cooper 12 minute run is one of the oldest and most popular fitness field tests and has been used by many people of all ages (see Table 3.2). Take this test if you are healthy, already participating in an exercise program, and doing exercise that involves running (e.g., jogging, tennis, basketball, volleyball).

Take this test on a 440 yard running track; you will need either a stopwatch or a clock with a second hand. Warm up with some easy jogging and stretching. The object of the test is to run as far as possible in 12 minutes; record the distance you traveled in miles using a decimal figure. For example, if you ran exactly 6 laps on a 440 yard track, you would have covered 1.5 miles. Check your fitness rating on Table 3.2.

6 Mile Bicycle Test

The bicycle test is appropriate if you have been riding a bicycle regularly for at least 3 to 4 weeks. Take this test on the bicycle you plan to use in your exercise program; the type of bicycle (e.g., 10-speed, mountain bike, 3-speed, cruiser) you use will affect

TABLE 3.2   Cooper 12 Minute Run

	Rating/Distance (miles)					
Men	*Very Poor*	*Poor*	*Fair*	*Good*	*Excellent*	*Superior*
Age: 18–29	<1.34	1.34–1.44	1.45–1.53	1.54–1.64	1.65–1.80	>1.80
30–39	<1.29	1.29–1.38	1.39–1.48	1.49–1.60	1.61–1.76	>1.76
40–49	<1.23	1.23–1.32	1.33–1.41	1.42–1.53	1.54–1.70	>1.70
50–59	<1.15	1.15–1.24	1.25–1.32	1.33–1.44	1.45–1.61	>1.61
60 and over	<1.05	1.05–1.14	1.15–1.23	1.24–1.36	1.37–1.56	>1.56
Women	*Very Poor*	*Poor*	*Fair*	*Good*	*Excellent*	*Superior*
Age: 18–29	<1.16	1.16–1.24	1.25–1.32	1.33–1.44	1.45–1.60	>1.60
30–39	<1.11	1.11–1.20	1.21–1.26	1.27–1.37	1.38–1.52	>1.52
40–49	<1.05	1.05–1.12	1.13–1.20	1.21–1.31	1.32–1.44	>1.44
50–59	<0.98	0.98–1.05	1.06–1.12	1.13–1.20	1.21–1.32	>1.32
60 and over	<0.94	0.94–0.98	0.99–1.06	1.07–1.17	1.18–1.34	>1.34

Source: From *The New Aerobics* by Kenneth H. Cooper. Copyright © 1970 by Kenneth H. Cooper. Used by permission of Bantam Books, a division of Random House, Inc.

your performance on this test. Regardless of which bicycle you use, the test is good for approximating your cycling fitness and useful for identifying your starting place.

Find a flat course where you can ride 6 miles without interference from automobiles or other bicycles. Although a bicycle track is preferred, it is unavailable to most people. A road with a bicycle lane and a park that does not allow cars are good places to take the test. Before taking the test, warm up by riding at a relatively slow pace for 4–10 minutes; then, ride the 6 mile course as fast as you can. Assess your fitness by comparing your time with the norms on Table 3.3.

TABLE 3.3   6 Mile Bicycle Test

	Time (minutes: seconds)				
Males (yr.)	*High*	*Above Average*	*Average*	*Below Average*	*Low*
18–29	<14:00	14:01–16:00	16:01–18:00	18:01–20:00	>20:00
30–39	<14:15	14:16–16:15	16:16–18:15	18:16–20:15	>20:15
40–49	<14:30	14:31–16:30	16:31–18:30	18:31–20:30	>20:30
50–59	<15:00	15:01–17:00	17:01–19:00	19:01–21:00	>21:00
60–69	<16:00	16:01–18:00	18:01–20:00	20:01–22:00	>22:00
Females (yr.)	*High*	*Above Average*	*Average*	*Below Average*	*Low*
18–29	<14:30	14:31–16:30	16:31–18:30	18:31–20:30	>20:30
30–39	<14:45	14:46–16:45	16:46–18:45	18:46–20:45	>20:45
40–49	<15:00	15:01–17:00	17:01–19:00	19:01–21:00	>21:00
50–59	<15:30	15:31–17:30	17:31–19:30	19:31–21:30	>21:30
60–69	<16:30	16:31–18:30	18:31–20:30	20:31–22:30	>22:30

12 Minute Swim Test

Use the 12 minute swim test if you plan to swim as part of your exercise program. You will need a swimming pool, a stopwatch, and a partner to time and count your laps. Before taking the test, warm up by swimming a few laps. The object of the test is to swim as far as possible in 12 minutes; it is best to swim at a steady pace. Check your fitness rating on Table 3.4.

Designing an Endurance Fitness Program

Start by setting goals. Do you want to exercise mainly to improve your health? Is your goal fitness for enhanced sports performance, or do you want to run, bike, or swim faster to gain a sense of individual achievement? Be honest with yourself, and set realistic goals you can achieve.

Basic Endurance Fitness for Health

The goal of the basic health-promoting fitness program is to do at least 30 minutes of accumulated physical activity per day. You do not have to do all the exercise at once—walking briskly to your car before and after work, mowing the lawn, climbing stairs, and completing several short workouts on a stationary bicycle can quickly add up to 30 minutes.

TABLE 3.4   12 Minute Swim Test

	Rating/Distance (yards)				
Men	*Very Poor*	*Poor*	*Fair*	*Good*	*Excellent*
Age: 13–19	<500	500–599	600–699	700–799	>800
20–29	<400	400–499	500–599	600–699	>700
30–39	<350	350–449	450–549	550–649	>650
40–49	<300	300–399	400–499	500–599	>600
50–59	<250	250–349	350–449	450–549	>550
60 and over	<250	250–299	300–399	400–499	>500
Women	*Very Poor*	*Poor*	*Fair*	*Good*	*Excellent*
Age: 13–19	<400	400–499	500–599	600–699	>700
20–29	<300	300–399	400–499	500–599	>600
30–39	<250	250–349	350–449	450–549	>550
40–49	<200	200–299	300–399	400–499	>500
50–59	<150	150–249	250–349	350–449	>450
60 and over	<150	150–199	200–299	300–399	>400

Source: "Swimming test," from *The Aerobics Program for Total Well-Being* by Kenneth H. Cooper M.D., M.P.H. Copyright © 1982 by Kenneth H. Cooper. Used by permission of Bantam Books, a division of Random House, Inc.

Try to be more active in everything you do. For example, when shopping, park farther from the grocery store. Instead of searching for a spot next to the front door, park in the back of the parking lot, and take a short walk to the store. Wash your car by hand instead of running it through the car wash. Take your dog for a walk every night (dogs benefit from exercise, too). In short, move more and sit less. Table 3.5 shows how you can increase your fitness by doing ordinary activities.

You will likely achieve your goal of 30 minutes of activity a day if you schedule a time for exercise every day. Until recently, health experts said that for exercise to benefit your health, you need to exercise vigorously for 20 to 60 minutes 3 to 5 days per week (ACSM, 1998). Although that is a desirable goal, you can still benefit from much less activity. However, given human nature, most people will not devote even 30 minutes a day to physical activity unless it is scheduled. Therefore, to ensure that you accomplish your endurance fitness goals, consider setting aside a specific time for a daily walk, run, or swim.

A useful guideline to help determine the proper amount of exercise is the Activity Pyramid (Figure 3.1). Everyone should attempt to increase the activities listed at the base of the pyramid; try to become more active during your everyday activities (see Table 3.5). If you are following a structured exercise program, try to

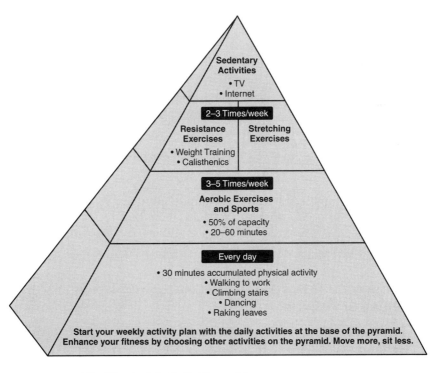

FIGURE 3.1   The Physical Activity Pyramid.

TABLE 3.5   Some Simple Ways to Be More Active

Bike to work	Plant bushes and trees
Carry a child upstairs	Play catch with a child or your friends
Clean the cobwebs from the ceiling	Play Frisbee
Clean the rain gutters	Play golf and do not rent a cart
Climb stairs instead of taking the elevator	Play tag with a child
Cross-country ski on the street when it snows	Rent a rowboat
Dig postholes	Ride a stationary bicycle during commercials
Do errands by bicycle or on foot	Run to catch a plane or bus
Edge the lawn	Run upstairs
Enter a charity walk-a-thon	Sand the deck (by hand)
Explore a new city on foot	Scrub the floors
Explore your city on foot	Shovel some snow
Go bowling	Sweep the walkway
Go dancing	Take a lunch-time hike
Go for a hike	Take the dog for a walk
Help out at children's soccer practice	Trim the hedge
Hit a bucket of golf balls	Vacuum the rug
Hit some baseballs at the batting cage	Walk around a large museum
Lay some cement	Walk fast
Make exercise bets ("twenty push-ups if you lose")	Walk to work
Make passionate love	Walk up some stairs
Move some furniture	Wash and wax your car by hand
Mow the lawn	Weed the garden
Paint the walls	

consistently do the activities in the middle of the pyramid. If you exercise faithfully, add variety to your program by including recreational sports. Everyone should decrease his or her sedentary activities, such as watching television, playing computer games, and prolonged sitting.

Endurance Program for Performance-Level Physical Fitness

The basic program contributes to your health and reduces your chances of getting heart disease. However, the basic program is not enough if you want to get into shape for your favorite sports or to control unwanted body fat. For this, you must go on a structured exercise program that carefully considers the type, duration, intensity, and frequency of exercise. Researchers have found that regular, vigorous exercise provides benefits beyond those provided by the basic, 30 minutes-a-day program.

Type of Exercise

The best sports and exercises for developing significant endurance fitness use large muscle groups repeatedly for at least 20 minutes; these include walking, jogging, cross-country skiing, swimming, and cycling. Soccer, basketball, and tennis also develop endurance if you are skilled and play them for prolonged periods.

Select exercises you can do regularly; do not choose cross-country skiing as your main form of exercise if you live in Florida and can only ski on vacation. If you like to run but live in a congested urban area where jogging is difficult or dangerous, perhaps you could run on a treadmill at a local health club.

Cross-training is a good training method for many people; it combines more than one type of endurance exercise in your program at a time. Including multiple exercises, such as swimming and running or stair-stepping and cycling, adds variety to your program. Also, it prepares you for a greater variety of physical challenges.

On the other hand, if you want to excel at any single activity, cross-training will hamper your progress. As with any type of movement, performances in endurance exercises are very specific. Adaptations (improved fitness) from running are different from those you get in swimming, cycling, or walking. In fact, training for one activity may interfere with your progress in another activity.

Intensity of Training

Significant improvements in endurance capacity occur when you train above 50 percent of maximum capacity (maximal oxygen consumption, $\dot{V}O_{2max}$). If you are a beginner or have low fitness capabilities, you can make progress initially training at 40–50 percent of $\dot{V}O_{2max}$ (ACSM, 1998). This intensity stresses your body enough to produce changes in the heart, lungs, circulation, and cells (e.g., increased heart pumping capacity, blood volume, and cell energy generation capacity). These changes improve your body's ability to transport oxygen and to use fuels to exercise.

You can use your exercise heart rate as a measure of your exercise intensity. A given percentage of maximum heart rate during exercise will approximately be 10 percent more than the percentage of maximal oxygen consumption (ACSM, 1998). For example, exercising at 50 percent of maximum heart rate corresponds to approximately 40 percent of maximal oxygen consumption.

To use heart rate as a measure of exercise intensity, you must first determine your maximum heart rate. Maximum heart rate is most accurately measured by a treadmill test conducted in a hospital or exercise laboratory. However, you can get a rough estimate of your maximum heart rate by subtracting your age from 220. For example, if you are 20 years old, your predicted maximum heart rate is 200 beats per minute (220 − 20 = 200). This technique approximates maximum heart rate; however, yours may vary from this considerably.

Estimate your training intensity by measuring your exercise heart rate. You get a significant endurance training effect when your heart rate reaches 55/65–90 percent of maximum heart rate (ACSM, 1998). This range of heart rates is called your *target heart rate* and corresponds to an increased metabolic rate that causes your body to improve its fitness. Use 55 percent as your lower value if you are extremely unfit and 65 percent as the lower value if you are physically fit and active. To calculate your target heart rate range, multiply your maximum heart rate first by either 0.55 or 0.65 (depending on your fitness) and then by 0.9. These two heart rates represent the upper and lower limits of your ideal exercise intensity.

You can measure your exercise heart rate by using a heart-rate monitor. Many companies manufacture these accurate, simple-to-use devices; prices range from less than $100 to more than $500. Yet, they are unnecessary for the average person (unless you like gadgets).

You can get a good estimate of your exercise heart rate by taking your pulse rate for 10 seconds immediately after you stop exercising. For example, suppose you are jogging around the neighborhood and have to stop at a red light. Take your pulse for ten seconds, and multiply the value by six to get your exercise heart rate. Based on this formula, if you count 20 beats in 10 seconds, your exercise heart rate is 120 beats per minute.

Do not worry too much if your exercise heart rate varies slightly from your target heart rate. As long as you are exercising at a vigorous pace that you can sustain reasonably for more than 20 minutes, you will improve your fitness. However, you will not progress in your program if you do not train intensely enough. Likewise, you may get injured if you train consistently at close to maximum intensity. Learn to *feel* the correct training pace. If you feel exhausted from training too intensely, slow down next time. If you feel that you are not tired enough, try working out a little harder.

Heart rate response to exercise is exercise specific—you cannot compare a heart rate achieved by swimming with one you achieved by running; the stresses of swimming, running, and cycling are somewhat different. You swim in a horizontal position but run upright. Also, water pressure triggers a reflex that slows down the heart rate. Thus, the same relative increase in metabolic rate achieved in these sports would produce a lower heart rate during swimming than cycling or running.

Two other simple techniques for assessing proper training intensity are *relative perceived exertion (RPE)* and *the talk test.* With RPE (Figure 3.2), you learn to associate a given exercise intensity on the RPE scale with how you feel during the exercise. In general, try to exercise at an intensity between 5 and 8 (strong to very strong) on the scale. The talk test can also help you exercise at an intensity that improves endurance, yet minimizes the risk of injury. This test can be taken while running or cycling but cannot be taken while swimming. In this technique, exercise at the fastest pace you can comfortably carry on a conversation, this will put you at approximately 70–80 percent of maximum heart rate—approximately your target heart rate (ACSM, 1998).

Training Duration

As discussed, you get benefits from even short exercise sessions lasting only a few minutes. However, significant improvements in endurance fitness occur with

Rating	Perceived Exertion
0	Nothing at all
0.5	Very, very weak
1	Very weak
2	Weak
3	Moderate
4	Somewhat strong
5	Strong
6	
7	Very strong
8	
9	
10	Very, very strong
•	Maximal

FIGURE 3.2   Ratings of Perceived Exertion.

sustained exercise workouts of 20–60 minutes. Continuous exercise is required to change your cell metabolic capacity. Although you can get good improvements by training very intensely for short periods (i.e., interval training), this training is uncomfortable and increases your chance of injury.

Training Frequency

As discussed, try to do 30 minutes of accumulated physical activity every day. However, intense training above 50 percent of maximum capacity should be practiced only 3–5 days per week. Training more frequently greatly increases the risk of overuse injuries and overtraining. Overtraining (an imbalance between training and recovery) can lead to chronic fatigue, suppression of the immune system, hormone abnormalities, and psychological depression.

Always remember the purpose of training; stress your body so that it adapts and improves its function. Sometimes rest is as important as intense training. The process of exercise training involves stress, followed by a recovery period in which your body becomes more fit. Without proper recovery, the body quickly breaks down.

Types of Training

OVERDISTANCE TRAINING. *Overdistance training* involves exercising for sustained periods. For the beginner, overdistance training might be a 30 minute walk, 5 times per week. A dedicated jogger might go for a 1 hour run, whereas a serious swimmer might swim 3,000 yards. Overdistance training for a cyclist might be a 25 mile ride to the next town. The cross-country skier might ski a 5–10 mile loop. People who are serious about overdistance training typically train 3–6 days per week. Training more frequently usually leads to overuse injuries; training less frequently can also lead to injury and is less effective for building high levels of endurance.

Overdistance training increases the mitochondria in your cells, which increases your metabolic capacity. These increases help you burn fats better, take in more oxygen, and protect your cells from chemical damage (i.e., free radicals).

INTERVAL TRAINING.   To increase pace and speed during endurance exercise, you have to practice interval training. *Interval training* involves performing repeated exercises at set distances or times. This training helps the body move at faster speeds by training the nervous system to react more quickly, increasing the heart's ability to pump blood, and helping the cells cope with rapid metabolism. Interval training builds aerobic capacity quickly; however, because of its high intensity, it is uncomfortable and increases the risk of injury.

You can use interval-training techniques for almost any exercise and even motor skills. For example, a middle-distance runner might do repeated bouts of 400 meter runs at 90–100 percent of maximum effort. The boxer might hit the punching bag for fifteen one-minute intervals with one minute of rest between exercise bouts. The swimmer might swim 100 meters at 90 percent effort for 15 repetitions with 3 minutes rest between repetitions.

The four components of interval training are *distance, repetitions, intensity,* and *rest.* Distance refers to either the distance or time of the exercise interval. Repetition is the number of times the exercise is repeated. Intensity is the speed of the exercise, and rest is the amount of time between exercises.

Each factor of interval training is related to the others. In general, the more intense the exercise, the fewer the repetitions, the more rest required. For example, a runner performing 400 meter runs at 100 percent of maximum intensity (speed) might manage only 4–6 repetitions. A person working at only 75 percent of maximum intensity might manage 8–15 repetitions.

Do not practice interval training more than three days per week; this exercise can be exhausting and easily lead to injury. Let your body tell you how many days you can tolerate. If you are overly tired after 3 days of interval training per week, cut back to 1 to 2 days. Likewise, if you feel good, try increasing the intensity or volume, and see what happens. The best advise is to begin slowly and progress conservatively.

Interval Training for Running.   Intervals range in distance from 15 to 50 meters for a football player or tennis player to several miles for a marathon runner. Keep in mind the desired outcome. If your goal is to develop peak speed and power, keep the interval distance short. On the other hand, if you hope to develop endurance for sustained efforts, then the interval distance should be longer.

For a beginning interval training program, run the straightaways at approximately 80 percent of maximum speed, and walk the turns on a standard 400 meter track. Start by doing two laps (800 meters)—running the straightaways and walking the turns. Build up gradually until you can do 8 laps (16 straightaways). As your fitness improves, sprint the straightaways at full speed; then, sprint the straightaways and jog the turns.

Graduate to 200 meter intervals as fitness improves. Begin by running two 200 meter intervals, and progress until you can do 8–10 repetitions. After each 200 meter interval, walk across the infield to the starting position. Because track races are run counterclockwise, you must change positions to strengthen both legs. In the 200 meters, you tend to put more stress on the inside leg (the leg closest to the rail of the track). If you run several 200 meter intervals, run some clockwise and others counterclockwise so that you develop your legs equally.

Finally, progress to 400 meter intervals; these can be extremely exhausting, particularly when run at high intensities. Again, start by running one or two 400 meter intervals. Then, build up until you can do 6–8 of them. Try to run each of the intervals in approximately the same time.

There are countless other variations of interval training for runners. You can run intervals up stairs (football stadium), up hills, and down hills. Tennis players can even do intervals running sideways. Defensive backs in football can do intervals running backwards, and soccer players can do intervals running zigzag patterns. The general principle for interval training program design is to examine the physical requirements of the sport and pattern the interval training program accordingly.

Interval Training for Swimming.   Interval training for swimming follows the same basic principles as running and cycling. In swimming, however, speed does not decrease with distance to the same extent as it does while running or cycling because the overall power output is less. As a result, the muscles can sustain a higher velocity.

The four variables in interval training for swimming are the number of swims, the distance of each swim, the speed of the swims, and the rest interval between swims. Interval distances are either 25 meters (one length of a standard pool) or greater. A typical interval training workout for swimming might be to swim ten repetitions of 100 meters (4 lengths of a 25 meter pool) with a 1-minute rest period between repetitions.

As with other forms of exercise, start slowly; begin swimming 25 meter intervals. As you improve your fitness, gradually add distance. For example, start by swimming five repetitions of 25 meters at about 90 percent effort. Gradually increase the number of repetitions to 10. After you achieve that level, increase the distance to 50 meters. Before you know it, you will be able to perform 10 or even 20 repetitions at 100 meters.

By manipulating the four variables (distance, speed, repetition, and rest), you can train your body for speed or endurance. Swimming longer distances at a slower pace will develop more endurance; swimming faster will develop speed.

Interval Training for Cycling.   You can do cycling intervals almost anywhere. With accurate odometers and heart-rate monitors available for cyclists, it is possible to pace interval training by time, distance, or heart rate.

With time intervals, you increase the riding pace (for example, increase your pace from 75 to 90 percent of maximum capacity) for a set amount of time. For example, suppose you are going for a 20 mile ride and want to do some intervals along the way. Ride for one minute at 95–100 percent of maximum, coast or ride easily for one minute, and repeat 5–10 times.

You can also do intervals at a set distance. Go to a track or park, and do intervals at a set distance. Typical interval distances might be 1 to 2 miles. Ride the distance at a predetermined percentage of maximum; then ride easy during the rest interval.

Like running, going up hills requires specific adaptation—if you want to be good at riding up hills, you have to train on hills. An example of an interval training program on hills might be to ride up a hill, then coast back to the bottom. Repeat 5–20 times (depending on the size of the hill).

Interval Training for Other Activities. You can practice interval training in almost every sport and exercise. For example, in tennis, you could hit against a wall or tennis ball machine for 2 minutes, rest 1 minute, and then repeat. On the stair-climbing machine, exercise for 2 minutes at a fast pace, rest 1 minute, and then repeat. In basketball, you could run 4 court lengths, shooting a layup at each end, rest, and then repeat. You are limited only by your imagination when setting up interval training programs.

Summary

Endurance is developed by training the cardiovascular system, metabolism, and muscle power. Endurance is very specific—building endurance in one activity does not fully transfer to another. The two principle training methods for developing endurance are overdistance and interval training. Build up gradually when practicing either technique.

Developing Muscle Strength

Muscle strength is an important fitness component for almost everyone. People interested in fitness for health reasons need strength to maintain healthy joints, strong bones, and metabolically active muscle tissue. Those interested in developing attractive, healthy-looking bodies do strength exercises so that they can have lean, shapely looking muscles. Sports enthusiasts, on the other hand, need it to make their movements forceful and powerful.

Increasing strength is quite simple—make the muscles work against increased resistance. You can increase muscle resistance using your own body weight, barbells and dumbbells, and weight machines, and you can build strength in your own home, a gym, or a weight-training class. You can even control the rate you gain strength. If you train intensely 3 to 4 times a week for 1 to 2 hours per workout, you will increase muscle strength and size rapidly. If you train 2 times a week for 30 minutes, you will make gains more slowly.

Principles of Strength Training

Resistance Exercise Methods

You can do resistance exercises four different ways—isometrics (exerting force against immovable objects), free weights (dumbbells and barbells), weight machines, and calisthenics (exercises that use body weight as the resistance). You can do isometrics and calisthenics almost anywhere, yet they are less effective than free weights and weight machines for gaining strength.

ISOMETRICS. Isometrics were very popular shortly after World War II, but they are less popular today. Unfortunately, you increase strength only in the joint positions you worked during the exercise. Several isometric exercises are available for the abdominal and neck muscles that are effective and can easily be added to your program. Several examples of simple, effective isometric exercises will be described in this chapter.

FREE WEIGHTS.   Most serious strength trainers prefer free weights because they are inexpensive, readily available, and easily adaptable to almost any movement or muscle action. Whole-body, dynamic exercises, such as the *clean* and *snatch,* are impossible using weight machines. These advanced exercises, described in Chapter 6, are popular with serious strength–speed athletes.

Free weights consist of barbells and dumbbells. Standard barbells come in a variety of sizes with the bar weighing 15–30 pounds. Weight plates for these barbells usually range in weight from 1.25 pounds to 25 pounds. Dumbbells are either adjustable or fixed. Fixed dumbbells, usually found in gyms and health clubs, range in weight from 1 pound to 150 pounds or more.

Most serious weight trainers use Olympic barbells, which are typically 7 feet long and weigh 45 pounds (20 kg). The bars are better balanced than standard barbells and are designed to hold more weight. Typical weight-plate configurations range from 2.5 pounds to 45 pounds. However, smaller and larger plates are also available for weight lifting contests. Athletes who do dynamic lifts, such as the *clean, snatch,* and *jerk,* often use rubber-covered bumper plates that do not damage the floor when dropped.

WEIGHT MACHINES.   Weight machines are the most popular resistance exercise devices for serious exercise enthusiasts. Machines are safer, easier to set up, more supportive, less difficult to use, and more comfortable than free weights. They also have high-tech appeal and do not clutter the floor with weight plates. Because weight machines are very expensive, they are usually available only in health clubs. Be careful when you buy weight machines designed for the home; inexpensive versions are typically poorly constructed and can be dangerous.

Weight machines come in a variety of designs that can be overwhelming to even an experienced weight trainer. Some incorporate variable resistance so that the resistance increases progressively throughout the range of motion of the exercise. Machines provide resistance by using weight stacks, weight plates, air, rubber bands, and hydraulic fluid. Some provide resistance during the active phase of the lift (concentric); others provide resistance during the active and recovery (eccentric) phase of the exercise. You can increase your strength on almost any weight machine if you exercise regularly and consistently.

CALISTHENICS.   Calisthenics are resistance exercises that use your body weight as resistance. They are excellent for a person who wants to develop muscle strength without joining a health club or devoting too much time to the activity. Table 4.1 lists some resistance exercises that require no equipment. If you are serious about increasing your strength, you should join a gym or health club; these facilities typically offer equipment beyond the scope of a home gym. Also, a gym gives you the opportunity to meet people interested in exercise.

Choosing the Exercises

Choose exercises that develop the major muscle groups of the body. Most people should select exercises that develop the shoulders, chest, upper back, arms, abdomen,

TABLE 4.1   Resistance Exercise Program without Equipment

Body Part	Exercise	Sets	Reps
Abdominals	Hip flexors	3	10–25
	Leg raises		
	Crunches		
	Sit-ups		
	Side-bends		
	Twists		
	Isometric tighteners	3	10–40
Calf	Heel raises	3	10–20
Deltoids	Push-ups	3	25
Latissumus dorsi "Lats"	Pull-ups	3	5
Lower back	Spine extensions	3	10–40
	Pelvic tilts		
Neck	Manual neck exercises	3	10–20
Thigh and buttocks	Squats	3	10–20
	Wall squats (Phantom chair)	3	10–40
Trapezius "Traps"	Isometric shoulder shrugs using low bar or doorknob for resistance	3	10–20

lower back, thighs and gluteals, and calves. This book suggests ten popular, well-known exercises; however, many other resistance exercises are as effective as the ones listed in this chapter. For a more comprehensive treatment of the subject, refer to my book, *Basic Weight Training for Men and Women*.

People interested in strength–speed sports (e.g., football, basketball, most track-and-field events, baseball and softball, soccer) should center their program around three primary types of lifts—presses, pulls, and multijoint leg exercises. Examples of presses include bench press, incline press, flat or incline press using dumbbells, standing press (military press), and seated press. Pulls include power cleans and snatches, squat or split cleans and snatches, dead lifts, and snatch and clean high pulls. Multijoint leg exercises include squats, leg presses, lunges, and step-ups. If you are interested in developing dynamic strength for sports, do these central exercises before doing auxiliary exercises, such as curls and sit-ups.

Frequency

As discussed in Chapter 2, you increase strength by making the muscles work against increased resistance. This stress is called *overload*. It is best to overload specific muscles 2–3 days per week. Most people choose 6–10 exercises and do them 3 times per week; others train 4 days per week (called a *split routine*), alternating between exercises for the upper and lower body. In split routines, you might exercise the chest, arms, shoulders, back, and abdominal muscles 2 days per week (e.g., Monday and Thursday), and your gluteal, thigh, and calf muscles the other two days (e.g., Tuesday and Friday).

Balance hard work in the gym with rest. Muscles increase in strength and size after the workout is over. You will not make significant gains if you do not allow your muscles to rest adequately between workouts. Sometimes rest is as important as hard work for improving fitness.

Repetitions, Sets, and Rest

Weight training programs are subdivided into repetitions and sets. Each time you complete the exercise movement, you do a repetition. In theory you could do almost any number of repetitions (one to thousands); however, in practice most people do 5–10 repetitions of each exercise. Each group of repetitions is called a *set*. Weight trainers generally do 3–5 sets of each exercise. For example, if you were doing 3 sets of 10 repetitions of the bench press exercise, you would perform 10 repetitions of the exercise, rest for 1–2 minutes, and then repeat the process two more times for a total of 3 sets.

The American College of Sports Medicine, the premier professional organization for sports scientists, recommends that beginners practice only one set of each exercise. According to recent studies, doing 1 set increases strength as much as doing 2 or more sets, but if you do practice only 1 set, make sure that it is high intensity (ACSM, 1998). The advantage of 1-set training is that you can work out quickly and have time for other exercises you enjoy. Practice more sets if you want to make faster progress or reach higher levels of strength.

The amount of rest between sets depends on your fitness goal. If you are trying to develop a combination of strength and endurance through resistance exercise, rest 1 to 2 minutes between sets. However, if your goal is to develop maximum strength, you may rest up to 5 minutes or more between sets. For these exercises, your goal is to exert maximum force during the exercise, an impossible feat if you have not recovered adequately from the last exercise.

Order of Exercises

If your primary goal is to gain strength, do large-muscle exercises, such as presses, pulls, and multijoint, lower-body exercises before doing exercises for smaller muscle groups, such as wrist curls and calf raises. Doing small-muscle exercises fatigues these muscles, causing them to limit performance when working on larger muscle groups.

Safety and Preventing Injury

Even experienced professional athletes often forget the primary purpose of exercise training—stimulate the body to improve its function. If you exercise improperly or overtrain, you will not improve, and you may get injured or become ill.

Do all of the exercises properly. Your back is extremely vulnerable to poor lifting technique. Observe the following principles when lifting any weight:

■ Lift the weight with your legs rather than your back. The muscles in your legs and butt are the strongest in your body; the muscles surrounding your spine are small and vulnerable.
■ Keep the weight close to your body when lifting so that you will lift the weight with your legs and hips rather than your back.
■ Keep your back straight and head level when picking up a weight from the ground.
■ Lift the weight smoothly from the ground.
■ Do not twist your torso when lifting a weight. This puts abnormal pressure on spinal muscles and discs.
■ Do not lift if you are so tired that you cannot use proper lifting technique. Lift within your capacity.
■ When using weight machines, make sure they are adjusted properly to your body. Sit properly so that your spine is supported.

WARMING UP.   Warm up before doing resistance exercises. Warm-up increases the temperature of muscles, which makes them work better and prevents injury. It also helps spread fluid (synovial fluid) throughout the joint, which protects vulnerable joint surfaces. Warm-up also helps to reinforce motor patterns (brain imprints that control movement) within the brain, which helps you perform the exercise more efficiently.

Do a few total body warm-up exercises, such as easy treadmill running, jumping jacks, or stationary cycling, before beginning your workout. Also, do some easy repetitions of each exercise before using maximal resistance. For example, if you plan to do heavy squats with 200–300 pounds, do 6–10 repetitions of the exercise with a light weight (e.g., 135 pounds) before attempting heavy weights.

BREATHING.   Breathing is very important for weight training exercises. Holding your breath and straining (called *Valsalva's maneuver*) will increase your blood pressure and may cause you to faint. In general, exhale during the active phase of the lift and inhale when returning to the starting position of the exercise. For example, for bench presses, inhale when lowering the weight to your chest and exhale when pushing the weight.

DECORUM IN THE WEIGHT ROOM.   Although being sociable is an enjoyable aspect of lifting weights, do not let it interfere with your progress or safety; be aware of your surroundings. Do not walk close to moving weight stacks or people doing lifts. Be particularly cautious around people doing dynamic lifts, such as cleans and snatches. Do not disturb people doing heavy lifts; you may distract them and cause them to either miss the lift or be injured.

SPOTTING.   Use an experienced spotter whenever you are doing a lift that could result in injury from a falling weight or missed lift. Spotters can also assist you during the lift, increasing the overall intensity of the exercise. They can help you complete a lift that you ordinarily might miss. If you are a novice, ask a fitness instructor to teach you proper spotting techniques.

COLLARS.   These devices hold the weights on the bar and should always be used when you lift. Without collars, weights can easily slip off the bar and injure you or others. Recently, collar clips of minimal weight were developed that are effective for keeping the weights on the bar.

CLOTHING.   Wear workout clothes that will not get caught in the machines or interfere with performance of the exercise. If you are doing leg exercises, such as squats, cleans, or snatches, wear shorts that will not tear during the motion. Shoes should be closed toed and provide good support during dynamic lifts. Women should wear bras that provide good breast support.

Weight lifting belts help support the spine and help maintain good posture during the lifts. Serious weight trainers often wrap their knees and wrists for additional support. Weight training can create hand calluses, so many people use weight lifting gloves to prevent them. Weight lifting supplies, such as belts, wraps, and shoes, can be purchased at sporting goods stores or through fitness magazines such as *Muscular Development* and *Powerlifting USA*.

Basic Weight Training Exercises

Exercises for the Chest and Shoulders

- Bench Press
- Standing and Seated Presses
- Upright Rowing
- Deltoid Raises

Exercises for the Upper Back

- Lat Pulls

Exercises for the Arms

- Biceps Curls
- Triceps Pushdowns

Exercises for the Abdomen

- Crunches

Exercises for the Thighs and Gluteals

- Squats
- Hamstring Curls

Exercises for the Calves

- Calf Raises

Literally hundreds of weight training exercises exist. The most popular exercises for the major muscle groups are listed in Table 4.2. This chapter will describe 10 of the most popular exercises that can serve as the basis for most strength training programs. The major muscle groups are shown in Figure 4.1.

TABLE 4.2   **Exercises for the Major Muscle Groups**

Body Part	Nautilus	Universal Gym	Free Weights
Abdominals	Abdominal rotary torso	Hip flexors Leg raises Crunches Sit-ups Side-bends	Hip flexors Leg raises Crunches Sit-ups Side-bends Isometric tighteners
Calf	Seated calf Heel raises	Calf press	Heel raises
Chest	Double chest	Chest press	Bench press Incline press

(Continued)

TABLE 4.2   **Exercises for the Major Muscle Groups** (*Continued*)

Body Part	Nautilus	Universal Gym	Free Weights
Deltoids	Lateral raise Overhead press Reverse pullover Double chest 10° chest 50° chest Seated dip Bench press Compound row Rotary shoulder	Bench press Shoulder shrugs Shoulder press Upright rows Rip-up Front raises Pull-ups	Raises Bench press Shoulder press Upright rows Pull-ups
Latissumus dorsi "Lats"	Pullovers Behind neck Torso arm Lat pulls Seated dip Compound row	Pull-ups Lat pulls Bent-over rows Pullovers Dips	Pull-ups Pullovers Dips Bent-over rows Lat pulls
Lower back	Lower back	Back extensions Back leg raise	Back extensions Good-mornings
Neck	4-way neck	Neck conditioning station	Neck harness: Manual exercises
Thigh and buttocks	Leg press Leg extension Leg curls Hip adductor Hip abductor	Leg press Leg curls Leg extension Adductor kick Abductor kick Back hip extension	Squats Leg press Leg extension Leg curls Power cleans Snatch Dead lifts
Trapezius "Traps"	Overhead press Lateral raise Reverse pullover Compound row Shoulder shrugs Rowing back	Shoulder press Shoulder shrugs Upright rows Bent-over rows Rip-up Front raises Pull-ups	Overhead press Lateral raise Shoulder shrugs Power cleans Upright rows

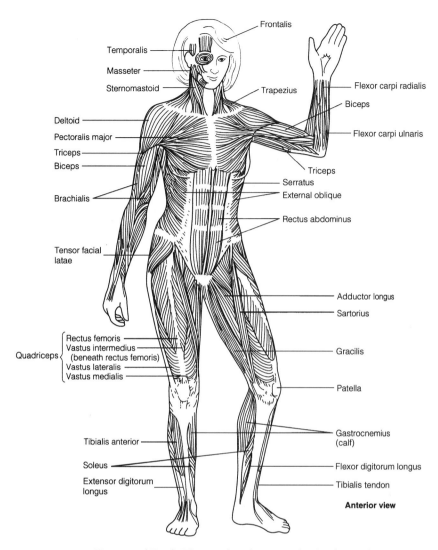

FIGURE 4.1a Front and Back Views of Major Muscles in the Body.

From *Basic Weight Training for Men and Women, 4th Edition* by Thomas D. Fahey. Copyright © 2000 by Mayfield Publishing Company. Reprinted by permission of the publisher.

Exercises for the Chest and Shoulders

The major muscles include the pectoralis major (chest), deltoid (shoulders), and trapezius (upper shoulder, upper back, and neck). Presses, such as the bench press and incline press, are best for developing these muscles; specific exercises that isolate specific muscles are also helpful. For example, fly exercises, which bring your arms across your chest, isolate the pectoralis major muscles (large chest muscle; one on each side).

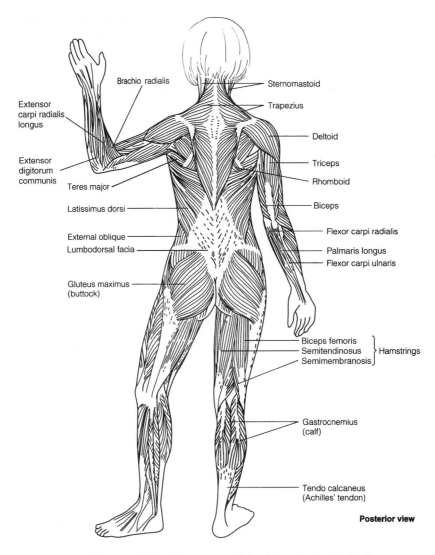

Brachio radialis

Extensor
carpi radialis
longus

Extensor
digitorum
communis

Teres major

Latissimus dorsi

External oblique

Lumbodorsal facia

Gluteus maximus
(buttock)

Sternomastoid

Trapezius

Deltoid

Triceps

Rhomboid

Biceps

Flexor carpi radialis

Palmaris longus

Flexor carpi ulnaris

Biceps femoris
Semitendinosus
Semimembranosis

Hamstrings

Gastrocnemius
(calf)

Tendo calcaneus
(Achilles' tendon)

Posterior view

FIGURE 4.1b   **Front and Back Views of Major Muscles in the Body.**

From *Basic Weight Training for Men and Women, 4th Edition* by Thomas D. Fahey. Copyright © 2000 by Mayfield Publishing Company. Reprinted by permission of the publisher.

Bench Press (Figure 4.2)

This popular exercise works the muscles of the chest, shoulders, and arms (pectoralis major, deltoid, and triceps muscles) using barbells, dumbbells, or weight machines. If you use a barbell, you should use a spotter and a bench with a built-in rack.

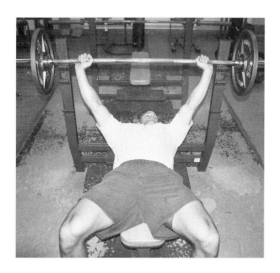

■ **FIGURE 4.2**

Lying on a bench face up with feet flat on the floor, start with arms extended and the weight over your chest, grasping the bar at approximately shoulder width. Under control, lower the weight to your chest; then push the weight to the starting position. You can also do this exercise with your feet placed on the bench. This position supports your lower back and better isolates the muscles of your chest, shoulders, and arms. However, you will not be able to lift as much weight.

Standing and Seated Presses (Figure 4.3)

This exercise develops the deltoids, triceps, and trapezius muscles. The standing or military press has been a popular exercise for many years. However, many people excessively bend their lower backs when doing this exercise, which increases the risk of injury to spinal muscles and discs. If done properly, standing presses are excellent exercises. Variations of the seated press include standing barbell or dumbbell press (military press), seated dumbbell press, and behind-the-neck press. Many weight machines are also available for doing seated and standing overhead and behind-the-neck presses.

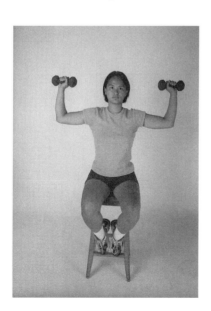

■ **FIGURE 4.3a**

Sit on a bench, preferably one with back support. Begin by holding the dumbbells at shoulder width.

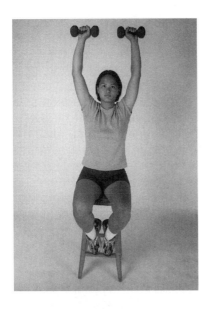

■ **FIGURE 4.3b**

Push the weights straight overhead, fully extending your elbows. Return the weights to the starting position.

Upright Rowing (Figure 4.4)

This exercise develops the deltoids, biceps, and trapezius muscles and is particularly useful for athletes who need strong neck muscles, such as football players, wrestlers, and martial artists. This exercise can be done with barbells or dumbbells in either upright or bent-over positions.

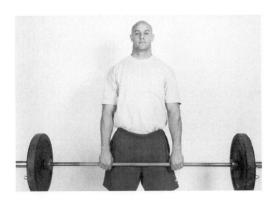

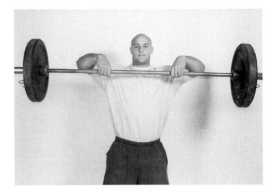

■ **FIGURE 4.4a**

Stand with your feet shoulder width apart, and grasp the bar in the middle with your hands approximately shoulder width apart and arms fully extended.

■ **FIGURE 4.4b**

Pull the weight upward until the bar reaches your collar bone. Return the bar to the starting position.

Deltoid Raises (Figure 4.5)

Deltoid raises develop your deltoids, the roundish muscles that form the shape of your shoulders. Because of the shape of this muscle, you must do this exercise to the front (anterior deltoid), side (lateral deltoid), and back (posterior deltoid) to develop all parts of it.

Front raises (anterior deltoid). Stand with your arms at your sides and your elbows extended, holding a dumbbell in each hand. With palms down and arms straight, raise your right arm until it is level with your shoulder in front of you. Lower the weight to the starting position, and repeat the exercise using your left arm.

Side raises (lateral deltoid).

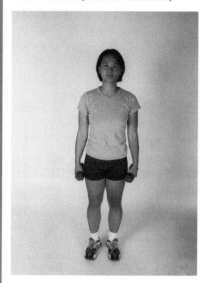

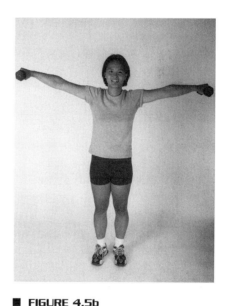

■ FIGURE 4.5a

Stand with your arms at your sides and your elbows extended, holding a dumbbell in each hand.

■ FIGURE 4.5b

With palms down and arms straight, raise your right arm until it is level with your shoulder to the side of you. Lower the weight to the starting position, and repeat the exercise using your left arm.

Back raises (posterior deltoid). From a standing position, bend at the waist. Stand with your arms at your sides and your elbows extended, holding a dumbbell in each hand. With palms down and arms straight, raise your right arm to the rear as far as possible. Lower the weight to the starting position, and repeat the exercise using your left arm.

Exercises for the Upper Back

The major muscles of the upper back include the trapezius ("traps") and latissimus dorsi ("lats") muscles. The upright rowing exercise, already described, is excellent for developing the traps. Pulling exercises, such as the clean and snatch, are also excellent and will be described in Chapter 6.

Lat Pulls (Figure 4.6)

This exercise requires a lat machine. Two basic types of lat machines are available—a freestanding machine that uses your body weight to stabilize you during the exercise and a machine with a seat that restrains your body with a seat belt or thigh support. If using heavy weights on a freestanding machine, you will need a spotter. Variations of this exercise include pull-ups and pullovers (machine or free weights).

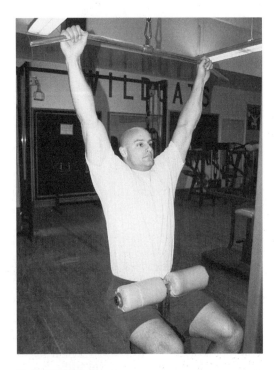

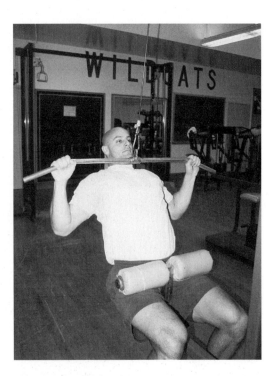

■ FIGURE 4.6a

From a seated or kneeling position (depending on the machine), grasp the bar overhead with your hands placed beyond shoulder width apart.

■ FIGURE 4.6b

Pull down the bar until it reaches your chest; be careful not to forcefully contact your neck to the bar because this could cause injury. Return to the starting position. You can also do this exercise by pulling the bar to the back of your neck rather than your chest.

Exercises for the Arms

Arm exercises are very popular with weight trainers. The two major arm muscles are the biceps brachius, which flexes or bends the elbow, and the triceps brachius, which extends or straightens the elbow.

Biceps Curls (Figure 4.7)

Do biceps curls with barbells, dumbbells, or biceps curl machines. Curl bars, which place your forearms at a 45° angle, are popular because they place less stress on the forearms during the exercise. You can also isolate the upper arm during the exercise by using special curl benches (i.e., preacher stand). Many other exercises also develop the biceps, such as lat pulls, pull-ups, upright rows, cleans, and snatches.

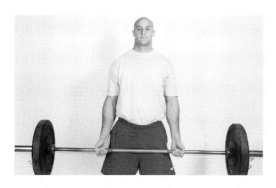

■ **FIGURE 4.7a**

Grasp a barbell at shoulder width with palms facing outward. Stand with your elbows extended and your arms against your body.

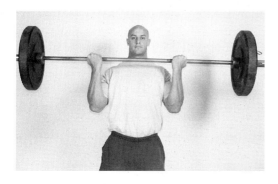

■ **FIGURE 4.7b**

Keeping your elbows close to your body, flex your elbows, and bring the bar to your chest. Return to the starting position. Use your biceps muscles to lift the weight; do not cheat by swaying your body.

Triceps Pushdowns

This exercise, which builds the triceps muscles (the muscles on the back of each arm), uses the lat machine. Other exercises that isolate the triceps and require barbells, dumbbells, and exercise machines are French curls and supine bench triceps extensions. Pressing exercises, such as the bench press, incline press, military press, and jerk, also develop the triceps muscles.

Stand facing the lat machine. Grasp the bar with your hands approximately 4–6 inches apart with palms facing your body. Fully extend your arms with your elbows held closely at your side. From this starting position, with elbows locked to your side, allow your hands to be pulled up to your chest; then firmly push the weight back to the starting position. If your elbows move during this exercise, you are cheating.

Exercises for the Abdomen

Abdominal muscles are very important for health, performance, and appearance. These muscles help stabilize the spine and prevent back pain. Trunk-twisting movements, which depend on strong abdominal muscles, are critical in sports requiring weight transfer, such as tennis, baseball, bowling, throwing (baseball, discus, javelin, hammer), karate, and boxing. Also, strong abdominal muscles are important for stabilizing the trunk in almost all movements using the large muscles of the body (e.g., running and jumping). Lean, toned midsections are prized as a critical part of a healthy, attractive-looking body.

Many exercises, such as crunches (shown here), sit-ups, slant-board sit-ups, trunk flexion machines, hanging knee raises, and twists, develop the abdominal muscles. A good exercise that you can do anywhere is the isometric abdominal exercise; periodically during the day, tighten your stomach muscles, and hold the contraction for 10 to 30 seconds.

Crunches (Figure 4.8)

Crunches are a variation of the sit-up, the traditional abdominal exercise. You do not need to do full sit-ups to develop fully trained abdominals; the abdominal muscles can get a tremendous workout by moving through a small range of motion. Crunches are as effective as sit-ups, and they place less stress on the back.

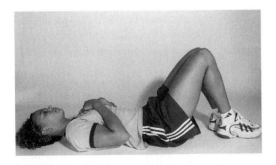

■ **FIGURE 4.8a**

Lie on your back on the floor with your feet flat on the floor.

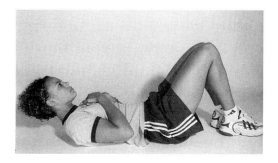

■ **FIGURE 4.8b**

With arms folded across your chest, curl your trunk up and forward by raising your head and shoulders from the ground. Your back should remain stationary. Increase resistance by holding a weight plate on your chest.

Exercises for the Thighs and Gluteals

Leg and thigh muscles are much more important for sports performance than arm, chest, and shoulder muscles. Yet, visit almost any gym, and you will see many people doing bench presses and curls and very few people doing squats and power cleans. If you want to improve your performance in sports in which you run, jump, or transfer your weight from back to front foot (tennis, golf, baseball, softball, boxing, etc.), do exercises that develop the large muscles of the legs and hips. Exercises for these muscles include squats, front squats, leg presses, cleans, snatches, lunges, step-ups, knee extensions, leg curls, jerks, push-presses, and calf raises.

The major muscle groups in the lower body include the quadriceps (quads—the muscles on the front of the thigh), the gluteus maximus (large butt muscle), the hamstrings (the back of the thigh), and the calf muscles (the back of the lower leg). The quadriceps and the hamstrings move the hip and knee joints. The quads extend (straighten) the knee and flex (bend) the hip. The hamstrings flex the knee and extend the hip. Exercises, such as squats and leg presses, that use the knees and hips work the hamstrings and quadriceps during the pushing (concentric) phase of the lift.

Other muscles cause your leg to move to the side (abduction and adduction) and are important for lateral motions. These can be developed on thigh abduction and adduction machines.

Squats (Figure 4.9)

You need a barbell and squat rack for this exercise. Many people like a squat rack with a safety platform to the side where you can rest the weight if you fail to complete the lift. Use 1 or 2 spotters if you are attempting near maximum weight. If you concentrate on this exercise, use a weight lifting belt and knee wraps. Also, during this lift, it is particularly important to use collars and to make sure the squat rack is adjusted properly for your height. Squats strengthen the quadriceps, gluteus maximus, hamstrings, and, to a certain extent, the calf muscles (stabilizers).

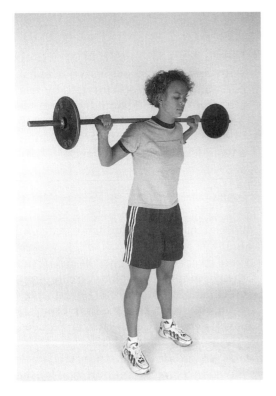

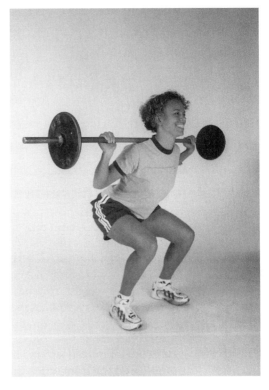

■ **FIGURE 4.9a**

Place the bar so that it rests on the fleshy part of your upper back. Grasp the bar with your hands for support. Some people like to put a pad on the bar to increase comfort. Stand with your feet shoulder width apart with your toes pointed slightly outward.

■ **FIGURE 4.9b**

Keep your head up and back straight during the lift. Squat down until your thighs are approximately parallel with the floor. Drive upward toward the starting position, keeping your back in a fixed position throughout the lift. Never bounce at the bottom of the squat—this could injure the ligaments of your knee.

Hamstring Curls (Figure 4.10)

You need a hamstring curl machine for this exercise. As discussed, you develop the hamstrings when you do squats and leg presses, but you can also develop these muscles with standing hamstring machines.

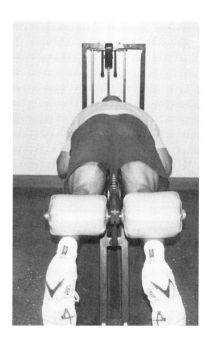

■ FIGURE 4.10

Lie face down on the bench with your heels under the pad. Make sure your knee caps are not touching the bench. Keeping your knees flat on the bench, flex your knees as much as possible, and then return to the starting position.

Exercises for the Calves

The two major calf muscles are the gastrocnemius and the soleus; these muscles plantar flex the ankle, which means they work when you lift your heels and go up on your toes. They are important muscles for jumping and running. You develop these muscles by putting weights on your shoulders, using a barbell or calf machine, and raising your heels off the ground.

Calf Raises

Using a calf machine, stand on your toes on the platform with your heels extending from the edge of the board and weight pads resting comfortably on each shoulder. Rise up on your toes, and then return to the starting position. As you gain strength, allow your heels to go below the level of the platform; this will increase strength and calf–Achilles tendon flexibility.

Basic Weight Training Programs
Countless variations of weight training programs exist. In this chapter, Tables 4.3 and 4.4 list basic and intermediate programs using the described lifts. Table 4.5 lists exercises for specific sports. Start with a general warm-up, such as exercising at an easy pace on a treadmill or stationary bicycle for 1–2 minutes. Do large muscle exercises, such as bench presses and squats, before doing smaller muscle exercises, such as biceps and hamstring curls. Do all the sets for an exercise before moving on to the next.

TABLE 4.3   Basic Weight Training Program

Exercise	Sets	Repetitions
Bench press	3	10
Seated press	3	10
Lat pulls	3	10
Upright rowing	3	10
Deltoid raises	3	10
Biceps curls	3	10
Triceps pushdowns	3	10
Crunches	3	10
Squats	3	10
Hamstring curls	3	10
Heel raises	3	10

TABLE 4.4   Intermediate Weight Training Program

Exercise	Sets	Repetitions
Bench press	5	5
Seated press	5	5
Lat pulls	3	10
Upright rowing	3	10
Deltoid raises	3	10
Biceps curls	3	10
Triceps pushdowns	3	10
Crunches	3	25
Squats	5	5
Hamstring curls	3	10
Heel raises	3	10

Note: Increase the weight during exercises using 5 sets of 5 repetitions.

TABLE 4.5   Suggested Exercises for Various Sports

Activity or Sport	Neck	Shoulders	Chest	Arms	Forearms	Upper Back	Lower Back	Abdominals	Thighs	Hamstrings	Calves
Badminton		✓	✓	✓	✓	✓			✓	✓	✓
Basketball		✓	✓	✓		✓	✓	✓	✓	✓	✓
Billiards		✓		✓	✓	✓	✓				
Canoeing		✓	✓	✓	✓	✓	✓	✓			
Cycling		✓		✓	✓	✓	✓	✓	✓	✓	✓
Dancing							✓	✓	✓	✓	✓
Field hockey		✓	✓	✓	✓	✓	✓	✓	✓	✓	✓
Fishing				✓	✓				✓	✓	✓
Football	✓	✓	✓	✓	✓	✓	✓	✓	✓	✓	✓
Golf		✓		✓	✓	✓	✓	✓	✓	✓	✓
Gymnastics		✓	✓	✓	✓	✓	✓	✓	✓	✓	✓
Jogging		✓		✓		✓	✓	✓	✓	✓	✓
Scuba diving			✓			✓	✓	✓	✓	✓	
Skiing, snow		✓		✓		✓	✓	✓	✓	✓	✓
Skiing, water	✓	✓		✓	✓	✓	✓	✓	✓	✓	✓
Squash		✓	✓	✓	✓	✓	✓	✓	✓	✓	✓
Swimming		✓	✓	✓	✓	✓	✓	✓	✓	✓	
Table tennis		✓		✓	✓	✓			✓	✓	✓
Tennis		✓	✓	✓	✓	✓	✓	✓	✓	✓	✓
Volleyball		✓	✓	✓	✓	✓	✓	✓	✓	✓	✓
Wrestling	✓	✓	✓	✓	✓	✓	✓	✓	✓	✓	✓

Source: From *Fit & Well: Core Concepts and Labs in Physical Fitness, Third Edition* by Thomas D. Fahey, Paul M. Insel, Walton T. Roth. Copyright © 1999 by Mayfield Publishing Company. Reprinted by permission of the publisher.

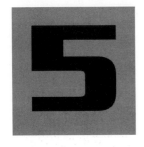

Developing Power and Speed

In sports, power is the ability to produce force rapidly, and it is the most important fitness component in strength–speed sports, such as tennis, football, soccer, basketball, most track-and-field events, field hockey, ice hockey, downhill skiing, golf, lacrosse, volleyball, and baseball. You move quickly and forcefully in these sports. How hard you hit the ball, how quickly you move on the court or field, or how rapidly and precisely you can apply force to the edge of the ski dictates the quality of your performance.

You also need power for endurance sports, such as distance running, cycling, swimming, and cross-country skiing. *Endurance* is the capacity to sustain a given exercise intensity. Except perhaps for marathon dancing (an event popular during the 1930s in which you danced until you dropped), there are no purely endurance events. Endurance sports consist of finite distances; the winner is the person who completes the distance in the fastest time, or the most powerful person over the contested distance. Although endurance is important, you need power as well in endurance sports.

This chapter describes exercises that develop speed and power for common total-body movements such as sprinting and changing directions on the court or field. Chapter 6 describes plyometric exercises that also develop speed and power in large lower- and upper-body muscle groups.

The Elements of Power

Power in sports depends on genetics, metabolic capacity (see Chapter 2), muscle size, skill, and nervous system capacity. With the exception of genetics, your training program must address each factor to maximize power for sport.

Genetics

Great athletes, such as Jim Thorpe, Wilma Rudolph, Michael Jordan, Mickey Mantle, Nadia Comaneci, Al Oerter, Willie Mays, and Muhammad Ali, were born with the capacity to produce great power when they moved. They are the geniuses of the sports world. Just as intellectual giants in the arts and sciences are born with great mental abilities, superstar athletes are born with their gift for generating power on the playing field. They had to train hard to become stars, but they started from a much higher level than the rest of us. Average people cannot expect to equal their physical prowess, no matter how hard they train. However, you can improve your performance in strength–speed sports if you systematically develop the components of power.

Metabolic Capacity

The metabolic basis of exercise was discussed in Chapter 2. To summarize, each sport relies primarily on one of the three energy systems—immediate, nonoxidative, and oxidative. Although all the energy systems are important to sustain life, specific sports tend to rely on one system more than the others. For example, weight lifters rely on the immediate system, 400 meter sprinters on the nonoxidative system, and marathon runners on the oxidative system. To maximize power, you must develop the energy system that sustains movement in your sport.

Muscle Size

Since the 1950s, athletes have weight trained to make themselves more powerful in their sport. Today's athletes are much bigger and stronger than those of 40 to 50 years ago—largely because of weight training. In the 1950s, it was not unusual to see 200 pound linemen in football; compare that with average weights for linemen of over 300 pounds on today's teams. Many of today's baseball players have forearms like Popeye; in contrast, pre-1960 players usually had very ordinary-looking muscles.

In women's sports, such as swimming, track-and-field, softball, volleyball, alpine skiing, and basketball, extensive weight training has produced athletes with well-developed muscles. Performance differences between men and women are largely due to differences in power output capacity; men can generate, particularly in the upper body, more force at a faster rate than women. Weight training has helped women narrow the gender gap in many sports.

A muscle's ability to exert force is largely determined by its size. Larger muscles have more tissue to contract, so they exert more force. However, in sports, the rate that muscles exert force is more important than the absolute force in determining sports performance. Although weight training is important for developing power for sports, it will not be effective unless you can learn to use your new strength in the sport. Effective strength (i.e., strength you can use in the sport) is determined by your nervous system's ability to control your muscles and the skill with which you execute movements.

Skill

Skilled performers make it look easy; they exhibit an economy of effort with little wasted motion. They concentrate all their forces into their movements and give seemingly flawless performances. The power produced by a National Basketball

Association (NBA) superstar dunking the ball, an Olympic discus thrower throwing over 200 feet, or a world-class ballet dancer jumping through the air seems beyond human capacity. These feats are possible because these athletes can precisely channel their incredible power into skilled movements.

Skill is the capacity to perform a specific movement. Skilled movements are orchestrated by your nervous system so that body positions and muscle contractions occur in precise sequences and speeds. The purpose of practice is to reinforce correct movements that result in more skillful performances, while eliminating inefficient or incorrect movements.

Skill is a prerequisite to successful performance in sports, regardless of your physical condition; you will not be effective in a sport if you have not developed skill. For example, a highly skilled Olympic gymnast would perform poorly on the golf course if he or she had not developed a good golf swing. Gymnasts must learn to control their bodies during the golf swing just as they had to learn to master movements on the balance beam or rings. Athletes in any skilled sport must direct most of their energies toward developing skill. Practicing the skill must never take a back seat to physical conditioning.

Many athletes mistakenly emphasize weight training at the expense of skill development. Strength gained in the weight room transfers slowly to the playing field. In fact, you can increase strength by 20–30 percent in the weight room and have absolutely no improvement in power in a sports movement. Only if you practice the skill will your movements become more powerful. Powerful, skilled movements depend on skill practice as well as conditioning.

Skill can overcome physical and conditioning deficiencies. Proper body positions, use of leverage, and timing can produce great force. Also, you are less likely to get injured when you move skillfully. Skilled movements depend on good movement postures, which place less stress on the bones, muscles, and joints.

TECHNOLOGY AND SKILL.   You live in a marvelous age for honing your sports skills. Even the average person, without the help of a coach, can use videotape and computers to improve technique in any motion. Yet, if you have a coach or sports expert to help you, all the better.

The procedure is simple. All you need is a home computer with video capture and a video camera. Video transfer capability is standard on many home computers, and inexpensive video transfer cards can be purchased for computers without this capacity. First, download a computer video clip of a sports movement from the Internet; these are widely available for any sport in both Macintosh and Windows formats. Next, take a video of yourself doing a skilled movement (e.g., hitting a tennis forehand, sprinting, or hitting a softball). Then, transfer the video onto your computer. Finally, compare your technique with that of the expert. A coach can point out important points.

Nervous System Capacity

As discussed in Chapter 2, your nervous system's ability to recruit or activate motor units (muscle fibers + nerve) is critical for generating power. Scientists have discovered that you can train motor units only if you recruit them, and the large, powerful motor units are recruited only during maximum powerful movements. If you want to train those motor units, you have to do maximum, explosive movements during your exercise sessions.

High-resistance weight training helps to recruit these difficult-to-train motor units. Doing high-speed training exercises and plyometrics also overloads the motor units that make you run fast, jump high, and throw far. Not only do you turn on these performance motor units but you also activate them longer, allowing you to sustain powerful movements during sports performances.

Similar to strength training, plyometric and speed exercises are effective for improving sports performance only if you also practice the skill. Research studies show that simultaneously practicing speed and plyometric exercises and the skill results in rapid improvement in sports performance (Delecluse, 1997). Strength training takes much longer to transfer to skilled movement. However, both weight training and speed–plyometric training eventually produce more powerful movements if integrated into a long-term, systematic program.

This chapter will describe basic speed and power exercises. When you combine weight training, general conditioning, and skill development, you are likely to improve your sports performance.

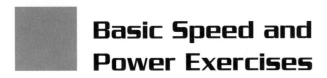

Basic Speed and Power Exercises

Sprinting

- Sprint Starts, Running
- Sprint Starts, Swimming
- Short Sprints
- Downhill Sprinting
- Speed Parachute
- Harness Sprinting
- Low Hurdles
- Stadium Stairs

- High Knees, Fast Arms
- Bounding Strides

Peak Power Training on the Stationary Bicycle

- Determining Optimal Frictional Resistance

Peak Power Weight Training

Sprinting

In sprinting, peak power occurs during the first 20–30 meters, and you can sustain it for only about 3 seconds before it drops off. In a sprint race, such as the 100 or 200 meter run, the winner is the person with the highest peak power output and the person who slows down the least at the end of the race.

In most strength–speed sports, critical movements last only a few seconds but require great power. For example, in football, plays seldom last more than 3 seconds. In tennis, you move from a ready position, set up for the shot, and then execute the stroke. Again, these critical movements take only a few seconds. In skiing, power applications occur when setting the edge; the remainder of the turn involves unweighting and setting up for the next turn. Baseball and softball players often exert great force when hitting the ball, baserunning, or making a play in the field. Movements in these sports are maximum and highly explosive for a few seconds; the rest of the time the players are mainly inactive.

When developing power for strength–speed sports, you need to enhance your capacity to accelerate (go from a stationary position to full speed in a short time) and to change directions rapidly. You can build these capacities with proper training and conditioning.

Technique is critical for powerful movement. When you are sprinting, either laterally or in a straight line, powerful movements depend on full extension of your legs and hips. The large muscles in the front and back of your thighs and hips are the strongest in the body. Use these muscles to their full capacity when you sprint, move to hit a tennis ball, or jump for a basketball. If you extend fully during powerful movements, you will run faster and jump higher than you ever thought possible.

Sprint Starts, Running (Figure 5.1)

These exercises are excellent for developing power and acceleration capacity in your legs. Figure 5.1 shows proper sprint-starting technique. The athlete in this sequence is a world-class sprinter. Notice the incredible extension he gets as he bursts from the blocks. Training to develop this explosive strength may carry over to other sports requiring power and speed.

When you are working on sprint starts, use starting blocks even though they are not absolutely necessary. If you are a football player, do sprint starts from the football stance. If you are a tennis player, soccer player, or baseball player, do some of your starts from the ready position for your sport. The ready position is your waiting position before you initiate a movement.

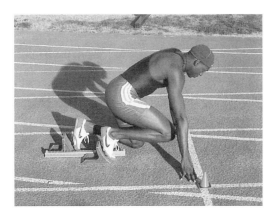

■ FIGURE 5.1a

"On your marks" position. Your feet are staggered 10–14 inches apart with your front foot placed approximately 20 inches from the starting line. Try to relax in this position.

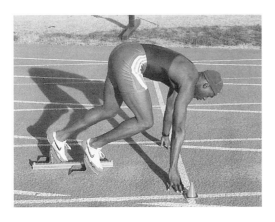

■ FIGURE 5.1b

"Set" position. Raise your back and hips. Your front leg bends about 90°, and your rear leg bends 120°. Right-handed people generally start with their left foot forward. Your back is flat, and your hips are slightly higher than your shoulders. You touch the ground with your fingertips, which raises your shoulders as high as possible. Do not put too much weight on your fingertips.

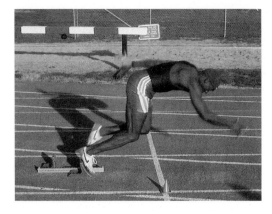

■ **FIGURE 5.1c**

"Go." Raise your shoulder so that you can direct force with your front driving leg through the length of your body.

■ **FIGURE 5.1d**

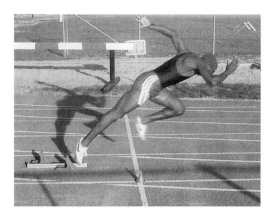

Drive the front leg fully so that your body forms a straight line from your hip to your heel. Push your rear foot hard against the block or ground as you drive your knee forward. As you drive forward, the arm on the side of the front foot drives straight forward, while the rear foot arm drives straight backward. Both arms are bent approximately 90–110°. Try to extend fully with your hips and knees, and drive your arms fully during the driving phases of the movement. After the start, run as fast as possible for 3–5 strides.

Start with 3 sprint starts, and progress to 10–20 starts as you increase fitness. After a few weeks, have someone time your starts so that you can gauge your progress. Also, videotape your starts to insure you are extending fully at the hips and knees.

Sprint Starts, Swimming (Figure 5.2)

If you are a swimmer, you can also develop acceleration capacity by working on starts. Starts are also beneficial for people who want to develop basic leg power and want some variety in their programs.

Modern starting technique uses an arc dive for entering the water. In this technique, the swimmer extends the body up and out. At the top of the arc, the swimmer bends at the waist so that he or she enters the water at a relatively steep trajectory. This technique allows the swimmer to travel farther over the water and to enter the pool more cleanly than a flat dive technique. If you are a serious swimmer, use the arc dive technique; however, if you are swimming for conditioning, it does not matter which technique you use.

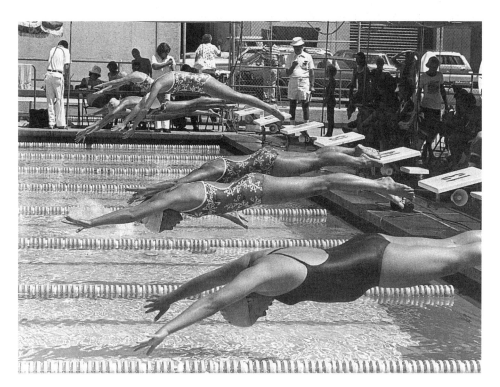

■ **FIGURE 5.2**

You can start from the side of the pool or a swimming starting block. Grasp the front of the block or side of the pool with head down and knees bent slightly. Pull against the block or poolside as you lift your head and flex your knees. Drive your body and arms upward and outward, fully extending the hips, knees, and ankles. If you are doing an arc dive, pike at the waist as you reach the peak of the dive. In the flat dive, continue to extend fully with the hips, knees, ankles, and shoulders. Enter the water as cleanly as possible by attempting to make the body enter the same hole in the water.

As with sprinting, do no more than 3–5 strokes after you hit the water. Start with 3–5 starts and progress to 15–20 as your fitness improves.

Short Sprints (Figure 5.3)

Short sprints, ranging from 20 to 50 yards, develop lower-body power and acceleration that will improve performance in most strength–speed sports. As with sprint starts, fully extend the knee and hip during the driving phase of the sprint movement. Powerful arm movement is critical to fast sprinting. Drive your arms forcefully in the direction you are going; do not flail your arms to the side.

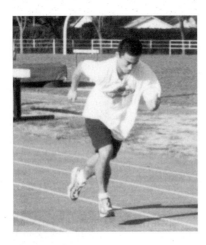 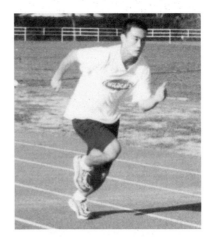

■ **FIGURE 5.3**

Start with longer distances (50–100 yards) at less than top speed. As your fitness improves, increase speed until you can sprint at 100 percent. Discontinue if you feel any pain or cramping in your muscles. Start with 3 to 5 repetitions with 30 to 60 seconds rest between sprints; gradually increase to 10 to 20 repetitions.

Proper technique helps you run faster with more power. Try to extend your hips fully during the push-off phase of the sprint. Vigorous arm action also helps you move faster and more powerfully.

Lateral sprint movements. These exercises are excellent for people interested in field sports, such as football, soccer, and field hockey. They also improve power in tennis, racquetball, basketball, and volleyball.

Using cones, shoes, or shirts, set up a zigzag course in which you run straight for 5 yards, run left at a 45° angle for 5 yards, then run right at a 45° angle. Another variation is to place two markers (cones or shoes) 10 yards apart. Sprint from the first marker to the second, touch it, and then sprint back to the first marker.

Backward sprinting. This exercise is excellent for people who must occasionally sprint backward in their sport (defensive backfield in football, basketball, soccer). Backward sprinting develops hamstring and gluteal power. Run distances of 10–50 yards, and progress similarly to short sprint exercises.

Downhill Sprinting (2–3 Percent Grade)

Sprinting downhill using a mild downgrade will allow you to increase your running speed and overload your fast-twitch motor units. This relatively new technique can improve your sprint speed rapidly. The Dallas Cowboys football team has a downhill track, which is made of Tartan (expensive material used in all-weather tracks), for developing sprint speed in their athletes.

Find a small hill that declines about 2–3°. A football field with a steep crown (higher in the middle than on the sides) is a good choice. Sprint 3–10 repetitions at distances ranging from 20–40 yards. Do not sprint down a steep hill (>5°) because you risk injury, and much of your energy will be devoted to keeping your balance rather than running fast.

Speed Parachute (Figure 5.4)

Speed parachutes, devices developed by Russian sprint coaches, also overload your muscles (fast-twitch motor units) during high-speed sprinting. You can purchase the chutes at track-and-field supply companies and at some sporting goods stores.

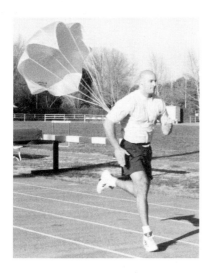

■ **FIGURE 5.4**

Attach 1–3 parachutes to the waist belt. Start with 1 and add chutes as your condition improves. As with short sprints, run 20–50 yards for 3–15 repetitions. Do not do parachute exercises until you have first run short sprints for 2–3 weeks.

A useful technique is to run 10–20 yards with the chutes and then release the chutes. This movement causes you to surge suddenly forward, which overloads your larger fast-twitch motor units.

Harness Sprinting (Figure 5.5)

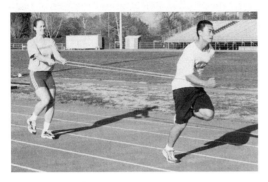

■ **FIGURE 5.5**

Harness sprinting is a variation of the parachute, and involves wearing a harness around your waist and pulling a weight sled or another person who is providing resistance. Vary the speed and resistance—the more resistance, the slower the speed and vice versa.

Low Hurdles (Figure 5.6)

Low hurdles (thirty-two inches) develop sprint speed and jumping power. Most high schools and colleges leave their hurdles on or near the track, at least during the winter and spring (track season); if hurdles are unavailable, use large cones or picnic benches. You can even use imaginary hurdles. If you use hurdle substitutes, make sure they will topple over if you hit them.

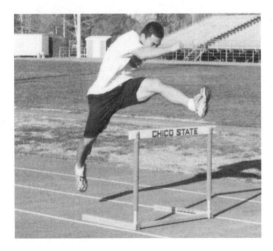

■ **FIGURE 5.6**

Set up 3 or 4 hurdles, on the grass or the track, 10 yards (8.5 meters) apart. The starting point is 15 yards (13 meters) from the first hurdle. Make sure that the hurdle supports face you; you want the hurdle to fall over if you hit it. In hurdling, you want to stride rather than jump over the hurdle. The take-off distance should be far enough away from the hurdle so that your leading leg sweeps forward and upward in a straight line; jumping too close to the hurdle causes you to jump over the hurdle. If the distance is too long, however, you will strike the hurdle. The stride across the hurdle must follow smoothly the normal sprinting stride and takes confidence, which only comes from practice.

The hurdling movement starts with a quick forward and upward thrust of the leading leg toward the hurdle. As you clear the hurdle, actively press your leg toward the ground. The trailing leg extends fully as you stride toward the hurdle. As you clear the hurdle, bend your knee and stretch it away from your body, and extend your opposite arm forward for balance. Try to take only three strides between hurdles.

Start off with only one hurdle. When you hurdle it with confidence, add more. When you can run the entire 3–4 hurdle course, start with 3–4 sets of hurdles, gradually increasing your speed. After you become proficient, run 6–10 sets of hurdles. Time your runs so that you can gauge your progress.

Stadium Stairs (Figure 5.7)

Running stairs is a tried-and-true technique for developing leg power; it overloads your body during the sprinting motion. The local football stadium is usually a great place to do this exercise; however, beware of old wooden football stadium seats that could collapse when you run on them.

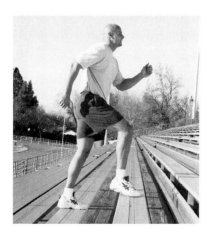 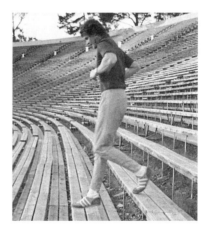

■ **FIGURE 5.7**

Find some unobstructed stairs that will support your weight. If you are using a football stadium, the number of repetitions will vary with the size of the stadium. Running up the stairs at a major university's football stadium will be much more difficult than at the local high school. As with other sprint exercises, start conservatively and build up the intensity and duration as your fitness improves.

Variations of stadium stair running include running two steps at a time, hopping up the stairs on one or two legs, and hopping up the stairs using a side-to-side motion, a good exercise for alpine skiers. Advanced fitness enthusiasts can increase the resistance by doing stadium stair exercises while wearing a weighted vest. These items are available at sporting goods stores and through track-and-field supply catalogs.

Be careful when running or hopping up stadium stairs, and particularly careful when going down the stairs. You can easily lose your balance and get seriously injured. Stop if you find yourself losing your balance or equilibrium. Also, this exercise may not be a good idea if you have kneecap pain; stair climbing, particularly going down stairs, produces a lot of pressure on your kneecaps. If you have kneecap pain the next day or several hours after running stadium stairs, cut down on your training volume, or eliminate the exercises from your program.

Stair climbing machines, although excellent for developing cardiovascular endurance, are less effective than running stadium stairs for developing lower-body power. When you run stadium stairs, you force your legs to extend vigorously during the push-off phase of the running stride and to absorb shock as you land; this movement develops dynamic strength in your legs that is not possible using stair-climbing machines, which require minimal stride length and little or no impact.

High Knees, Fast Arms (Figure 5.8)

This exercise develops sprint power and increases stride frequency, one of two factors determining sprint speed (the other being stride length). Do this exercise on a grass field or wooden gym floor to minimize impact.

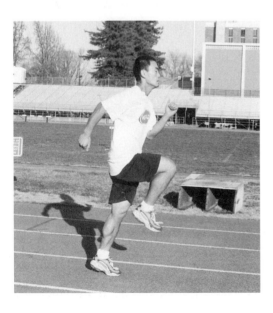

■ FIGURE 5.8

Simulating a sprint motion in a nearly stationary position, pump your arms and lift your knees as quickly as possible. Try to complete 20 strides in only 10 yards. Begin with 3 repetitions (3 sets of 10 yards). Progress to 10–20 repetitions.

Bounding Strides (Figure 5.9)

This exercise builds stride length for sprinting. Rather than taking many strides in a short distance (as in the high knee, fast arms exercise), you attempt to take as few strides as possible over a longer distance.

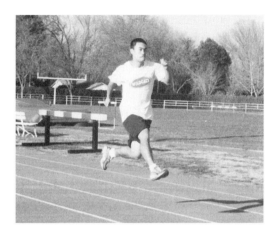

■ **FIGURE 5.9**

Do this exercise on a grass field or running track over a distance of 50–100 yards. Make your strides as long as possible, moving your arms vigorously in synchrony with your legs. Your strides should resemble bounding jumps. Begin with 2–3 repetitions and progress to 10 repetitions.

Peak Power Training on the Stationary Bicycle (Bicycle Ergometer)

The stationary bicycle is an excellent device for developing leg power. By training at peak power output, you can develop explosive strength in your legs that will carry over to other sports, and you will build the energy systems important in strength–speed sports.

Power on a stationary bicycle is a combination of pedal revolutions (rpm) and resistance (i.e., frictional resistance measured in kiloponds, or kp). Achieving peak power output requires that you establish the optimum combination of kiloponds and rpm. Too much resistance will decrease power output because your rpm's will be low. Likewise, if the resistance is too low, power will also be low because your capacity for increasing pedaling speed is limited.

Determining Optimal Frictional Resistance

To determine optimal frictional resistance for stationary bicycling power training (Table 5.1), first find a bicycle ergometer that allows you to adjust the frictional resistance (e.g., the Monark and Tunturi cycle ergometers). Set the frictional resistance on the bicycle at 1 kp. Warm up by pedaling at an easy pace for approximately 2 minutes. Then, ride as fast as you can for 30 seconds, and count the pedal revolutions. Every time your right leg extends, you have completed one pedal revolution. Multiply the pedal revolutions by

1; the result is your power index. Rest for 5 minutes, and then repeat the procedure using 2 kp. This time, multiply the pedal revolutions by 2. Rest for 5 minutes, and repeat using 3 kp. Repeat the procedure until the product of pedal revolutions starts to decrease, and then select the kilopond setting that produces the highest power rating. In this example, power output decreased when the frictional resistance increased from 3 to 4 kp. So, to produce the highest power rating, you would choose 3 or 3.5 kp as the friction for your power rides.

Set the kiloponds at the maximum power setting, and sprint as quickly as possible for 30 seconds. Begin with 3–5 sets of 30 seconds. As fitness improves, build up to 10–15 sets of 30 second sprints. Rest 3–5 minutes between sets.

Use this technique to develop power for time intervals ranging from 10 seconds to 10 minutes. The principle is the same. Count the pedal revolutions for the desired exercise time. The longer the time interval, the lower the kilopond setting will be. For longer time intervals, your goal is to maintain a given power output.

TABLE 5.1   Example of Procedure for Determining Peak Power

kp setting	Maximum revolutions in 30 seconds	Power rating
1	60	60
2	57	114
3	48	144
4	30	120

Peak Power Weight Training

You can also use the peak power training technique with weight training. The principle is the same as for the stationary bicycle. Calculate your peak power output for 5 repetitions of an exercise.[1] In general, use a weight that is 50–60 percent of the maximum weight you can lift for 1 repetition. Time how long it takes you to do 5 repetitions; do the lift as rapidly as possible. You must use good lifting technique throughout this training exercise.

Calculate the peak power workout weight for your lift. The following example is for the bench press (Table 5.2). In this example, the lifter can bench press 300 pounds for one repetition. For your program, begin with a weight

[1]Power is calculated by multiplying rpm, frictional resistance, and the distance the flywheel travels per revolution. Although the method cited here does not calculate power, it provides a useful index that is easy to understand.

that is 40–45 percent of your best 1-rep lift. You should use a rubber b
pad on the bar to protect yourself from injury. Next, time how long it ta
to bench press 5 reps, lifting the weight as rapidly as possible. Do not che
on the lift; go all the way down and all the way up. Then, repeat this procedure for weights that are 50, 60, and 70 percent of your 1-rep maximum
bench press. Your workout weight will be the one that renders the highest
pounds per second.

TABLE 5.2 Calculating Training Weight for Peak Power Training

1 rep max bench press = 300 lbs.

Percent max	Weight (lb)	Reps	Total weight for 5 reps (lb)	Time to complete 5 reps	Weight per second (total weight/time)
45	135	5	675	4.5	150
50	150	5	750	4.8	156.3 ⇐ peak power
60	180	5	900	6	150
70	210	5	1050	8.5	123.5

In this example, peak power output was at 50 percent of maximum. Your
workout weight should be 150–170 pounds. Do 3–5 sets of 5 repetitions at that
weight, pushing the weight as quickly as possible. Increase your weight when you
can do your sets in less than 5–6 seconds. This highly effective training technique
can produce rapid gains in strength and power.

Integrating Power Training into Your Workouts
Power training requires you to exercise at maximum intensity, which is
the only way to overload the large, fast motor units. This training is effective and will improve your power in sports, provided you also practice the skill. Because this training is high intensity, there is a higher risk
of injury and an easier chance of becoming overtrained. Overtraining is
an imbalance between training and recovery. You get overtrained when
you do not give yourself enough rest between workouts or you work out
too hard.
    Start gradually and progress slowly. Choose one or two of these ex-
ercises, and add more as you get in better shape. Gauge the appropri-
ateness of your workouts by how you feel the next day; if you are
extremely sore for one or two days after a power workout, then you have
done too much. In other words, listen to your body. Sample workouts
are described in Chapter 8.

Jumping and Plyometrics

Jumping exercises and plyometrics enhance performance in strength–speed sports because they increase leg power and train the nervous system to activate large muscle groups quickly when you move. Although the exercises described in Chapter 5 do improve your physical fitness for strength–speed sports, the exercises in this chapter enhance your capacity for single, explosive movements, such as jumping and hitting a golf or tennis ball.

Plyometric exercises involve rapid stretching then shortening of a muscle group during highly dynamic movements. The stretching causes a stretch reflex and an elastic recoil in your muscles, which when combined with a vigorous muscle contraction creates great force that overloads the muscles and increases strength and power.

Calf jumps are simple plyometric exercises in which you jump in place repeatedly using mainly your calf muscles. As you land on the ground after the first jump, you stretch your calf muscles to control your landing. The recoil from the stretch adds to the force of the muscle contraction used for the next jump.

The basic principle for all jumping and plyometric exercises is to absorb the shock with your arms or legs and then immediately to contract your muscles. For example, if you are doing a series of squat jumps, as soon as you land after one jump, jump again as quickly as possible. The more quickly you jump, the more you overload your muscles. These exercises train your nervous system to react quickly.

In untrained people, the nervous system reacts slowly when turning on the muscles during repeated muscle contractions (e.g., calf jumping). This protective reflex is designed to protect the legs from injury. With conditioning, you can train the nervous system to react more quickly and to activate leg muscles rapidly because stronger muscles and joints no longer need the protection of the reflex.

Jumping and plyometric exercises can cause great stress to your muscles, bones, and joints. All exercises in this chapter are considered moderate to high impact, so progress slowly. Do not do these exercises more than 2–3 days per week. If you feel pain in your muscles and joints for hours or days after a workout, modify your program or stop doing the exercises that give you trouble.

This chapter begins with simple, relatively low-impact exercises; more difficult exercises are presented later in the chapter. Do not attempt advanced exercises until you are in good condition and can do the exercises without pain. Start off by doing 1–2 sets of about 3–4 exercises. As you become better conditioned, build up to 3 sets of 6–10 exercises. Chapter 8 presents sample programs for people with various physical fitness goals.

Basic Jumping and Plyometric Exercises

Stationary Plyometrics

- Calf Jumps
- Rope Skipping
- Squat Jumps
- Tuck Squat Jumps
- Mule Kick Squat Jumps
- 360° Squat Jumps
- Pike Jumps
- One-Leg Squat Jumps
- Ice Skaters
- Lunge Jumps

Horizontal Jumps and Hops

- Standing Long Jumps
- Multiple Standing Long Jumps
- Standing Triple Jump
- Skiers
- Four Squares
- Cone Hops
- Hurdle Hops

Bounce Push-Ups

- Wall Bounce Push-Ups

- Floor Bounce Push-Ups

Box Jumping

- Step Downs
- Standing Long Jumps from a Box
- Ski Box Jumps
- Single-Leg Jump-Ups

Medicine Ball Exercises

- Play Catch with Yourself
- Medicine Ball or Shot Put Throws

Medicine Ball Exercises with a Partner

- Chest Passes
- Overhead Passes
- Medicine Ball Sit-Ups

Olympic Weight Lifting

- Power Clean
- Power Snatch
- Jerk

Stationary Plyometrics

Start with these simple exercises before progressing to movements that place more stress on your muscles and joints. With these exercises, you jump to and from the same place on the ground. More advanced exercises will progress to repeated distance jumps and finally to box jumps.

Calf Jumps (Figure 6.1)

This basic exercise develops jumping power in your calf muscles and is an excellent beginning exercise.

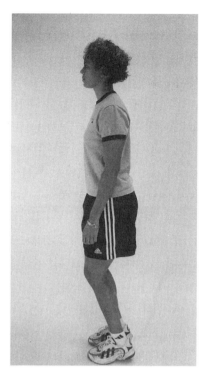

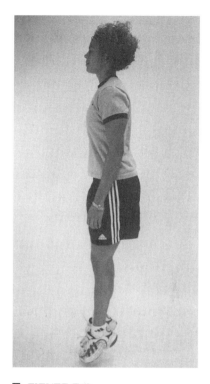

■ **FIGURE 6.1a**

Stand with your feet shoulder width apart and your hands on your hips. Bend your knees slightly.

■ **FIGURE 6.1b**

Using mainly your calf muscles, jump rapidly in place for 10 repetitions.

Variations: Advanced variations of this exercise include calf jump spins and one-leg calf jumps. With calf jump spins, attempt to spin as you jump, eventually going 360° between jumps. Do one-leg calf jumps the same way you do two-leg jumps except lift one leg off the ground when doing the exercise.

Rope Skipping (Figure 6.2)

Rope skipping is essentially the same as calf jumping, only more vigorous. This exercise conditions the nonoxidative energy system and develops jumping power, particularly in the calf muscles. Do this exercise using either boxer or playground style. In boxer style, you use a short rope and jump by yourself. In playground style, two people swing the rope while a third person jumps. For most people, boxer style is most practical.

Good jump ropes can be purchased at almost any sporting goods store. The best ones are made of leather, wooden handles, and ball-bearing swivels. With these swivels, the rope turns easily in the hand without tangling. Buy a rope that you can turn without hunching over during the exercise.

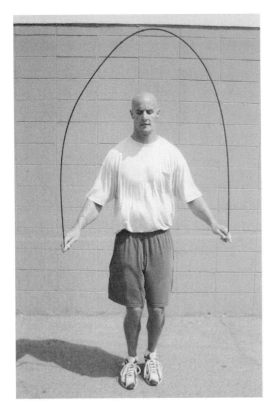

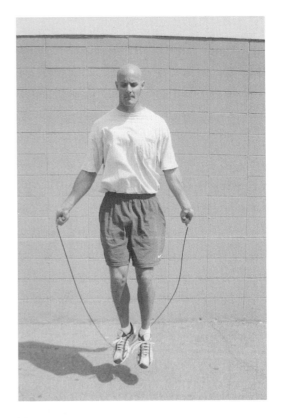

 FIGURE 6.2a

Hold one handle in each hand with the rope behind you. Swing the rope over your head.

FIGURE 6.2b

Jump over the rope when it reaches your feet. Continue swinging the rope and jumping over it. Speed up the tempo as your skill improves. Start with 5–10, 15 second segments and progress to 5–20, 1–3 minute segments.

As your skill improves, learn some of the many rope skipping variations, such as crossing your hands in front as you jump the rope and swinging the rope for 2 revolutions between jumps. You can also vary your foot movements so that they resemble running or dancing. Using a heavy rope or wearing a weighted vest increases the conditioning effect of rope skipping.

Squat Jumps (Figure 6.3)

These exercises are similar to calf jumps except that you bend your knees and squat between jumps. This basic exercise improves jumping power and is an important part of any plyometric program.

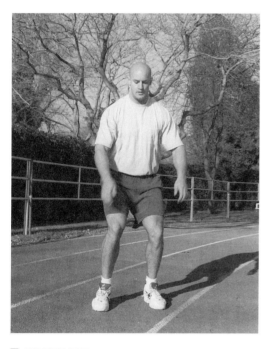

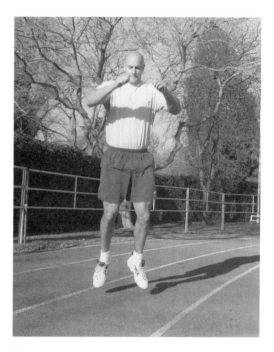

■ FIGURE 6.3a

Stand with your feet shoulder width apart, and bend your knees slightly.

■ FIGURE 6.3b

Jump up and drive your arms upward. As you land, retract your arms and squat down; then jump again as quickly and explosively as possible. Do 5–10 repetitions per set.

Tuck Squat Jumps (Figure 6.4)

Similar to squat jumps, these exercises are more vigorous. You have to jump higher off the ground to perform the knee tuck and still achieve a balanced landing.

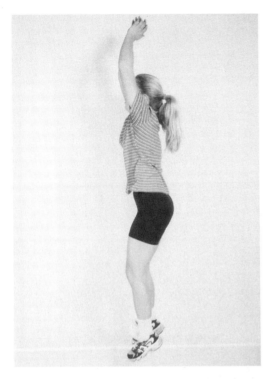

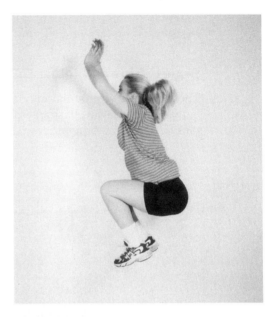

■ FIGURE 6.4b

Tuck your knees underneath you as you reach the height of the jump. As you land, extend your legs, retract your arms, and prepare to jump again. Do 5–10 repetitions, taking as little time as possible between jumps.

■ FIGURE 6.4a

Stand with your feet shoulder width apart, and bend your knees slightly. Jump up and drive your arms upward.

Mule Kick Squat Jumps (Figure 6.5)

This exercise is another variation of squat jumps.

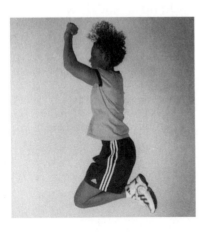

■ FIGURE 6.5

Stand with your feet shoulder width apart, and bend your knees slightly. Jump up and drive your arms upward. As you reach the top of the jump, kick your heels backward and touch the back of your thighs. As you land, extend your legs, retract your arms, and prepare to jump again. Do 5–10 repetitions, taking as little time as possible between jumps.

360° Squat Jumps (Figure 6.6)

This exercise is another variation of squat jumps and is similar to the 360° calf jumps described earlier, but it requires more fitness than most squat jumps. Start with 45–90° turns, and progress to 360° turns.

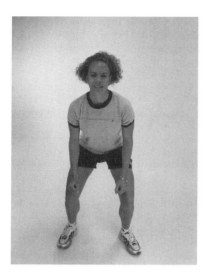

■ FIGURE 6.6a

Stand with your feet shoulder width apart, and bend your knees slightly.

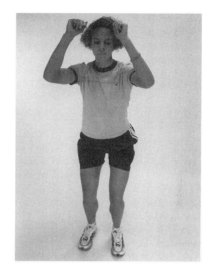

■ FIGURE 6.6b

Jump up and drive your arms upward.

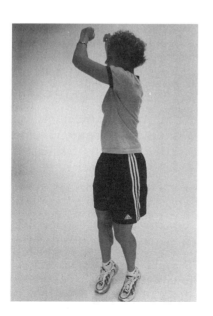

■ FIGURE 6.6c

Spin in the air as much as possible. As you land, retract your arms, and prepare to jump again. Start by rotating in only one direction. As you become more advanced, rotate to the left on one repetition and to the right on the next. Do 5–10 repetitions, taking as little time as possible between jumps. Advanced variations of this exercise include tuck and mule kick 360s.

Pike Jumps (Figure 6.7)

This advanced exercise requires superior jumping and power output capacity.

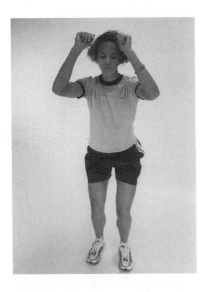

■ **FIGURE 6.7a**

Stand with your feet shoulder width apart, and bend your knees slightly.

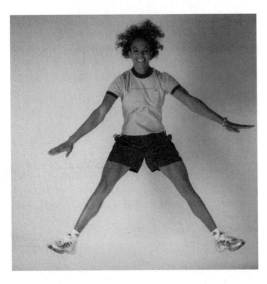

■ **FIGURE 6.7b**

Jump up and drive your arms upward. As you reach the top of the jump, extend your legs outward in a split position. As you land, retract your legs and arms, and prepare to jump again. Do 3–10 repetitions, taking as little time as possible between jumps.

One-Leg Squat Jumps (Figure 6.8)

Do not do these until you have conditioned your legs with two-leg squat jumps. Progress slowly; if you feel ankle, knee, or hip pain after doing this exercise, cut down on the volume, or eliminate it from your program.

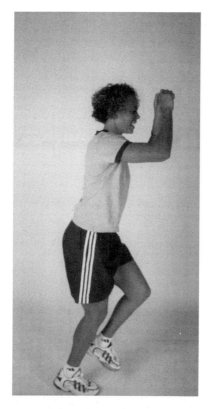

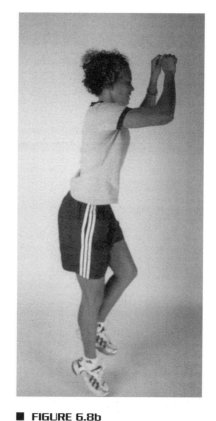

■ **FIGURE 6.8a**

Stand on one leg, and bend your knee slightly.

■ **FIGURE 6.8b**

Jump up and drive your arms upward. As you land, retract your arms, and immediately jump again. Do 5–10 repetitions, taking as little time as possible between jumps.

Variations (all advanced): one-leg tuck squat jumps, one-leg mule kick squat jumps, one-leg 360° squat jumps.

Ice Skaters (Figure 6.9)

This exercise develops the thigh muscles for lateral movements and stabilizes the spinal muscles for dynamic movements. Make sure to use shoes that give good traction, and choose an area that will give good footing.

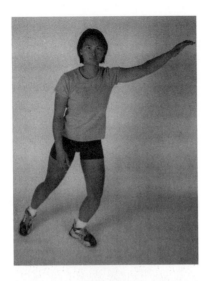

■ **FIGURE 6.9a**

Stand with your weight on the inside part of your feet.

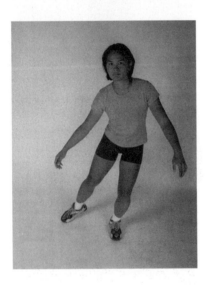

■ **FIGURE 6.9b**

Using a speed skating motion, drive off your left leg and swing both arms to the right; then immediately drive with the right leg to the left. Move as quickly as possible when going from one leg to the other.

Variations: *Sand ice skaters.* Do the ice skater exercise in the sand. This is a good way to begin doing this exercise because it is less stressful to the knee, hip, and ankle joints. Another variation is to use angled boxes. These wedge-shaped boxes allow better footing during the push-off phase and are popular with skaters and skiers. You can also practice ice skaters on a slide board. Slide boards are available commercially or can be manufactured cheaply using a piece of Formica and 2 × 4's.

Lunge Jumps (Figure 6.10)

The lunge or split jump builds your thigh, gluteal, and back muscles and develops your striding power for sprinting and lower-body flexibility.

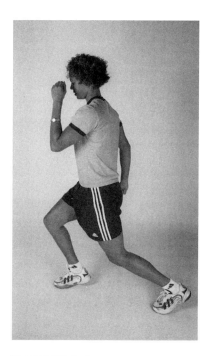

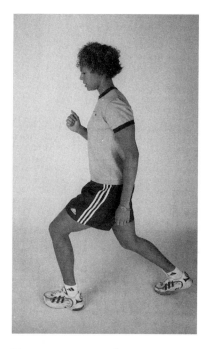

■ **FIGURE 6.10a**

From a standing position, jump up and then land in a split position with your right leg bent and your left leg extended in back of you.

■ **FIGURE 6.10b**

After you land, immediately jump up and again land in a split position with your legs reversed. One repetition occurs when each leg has been in the forward position. During this exercise, try to keep your body straight and to jump up as high as possible.

Horizontal Jumps and Hops

These more advanced exercises involve jumping and hopping horizontally. They develop basic leg power for jumping and running.

Standing Long Jumps (Figure 6.11)

In addition to increasing basic leg power, this exercise will help you gauge your progress. Measure your standing long jump every few weeks. If you do speed and plyometric exercises regularly, you will be amazed at how rapidly you improve.

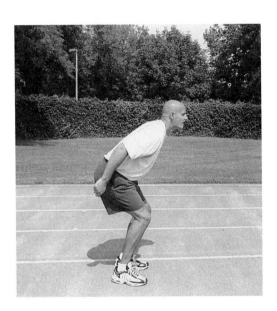
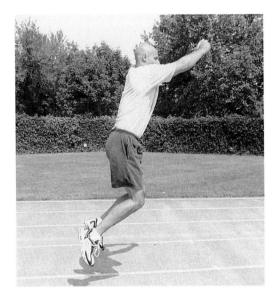

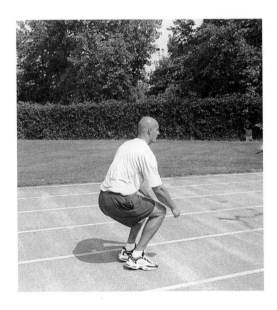

■ **FIGURE 6.11a–c**

Stand with your feet shoulder width apart and your toes just behind the starting (scratch) line. Bend your knees, and bring your hands below your waist. Then jump as far as you can. Try to extend fully with your ankles, knees, hips, and arms to jump as far as possible.

Multiple Standing Long Jumps
(Hops, Figure 6.12)

This is similar to the last exercise except that you take three jumps in succession.

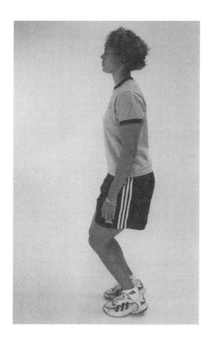

■ **FIGURE 6.12a**

Stand with your feet shoulder width apart and your toes just behind the starting (scratch) line. Bend your knees, and bring your hands below your waist.

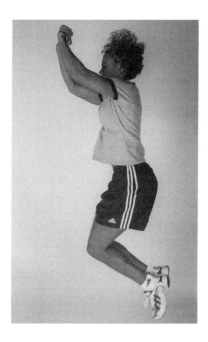

■ **FIGURE 6.12b**

Then jump as far as you can, extending fully with your ankles, knees, hips, and arms. As soon as you land, try to jump again as soon as possible. Repeat until you have jumped three times.

Standing Triple Jump (Figure 6.13)

The triple jump, formerly known as the *hop, step, and jump* because of its basic movements, can be seen in track-and-field competitions.

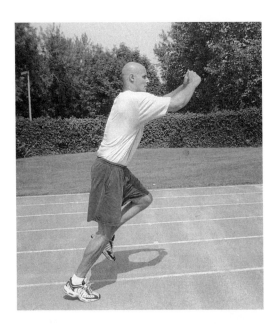

■ **FIGURE 6.13a**

Stand with your feet shoulder width apart and your toes just behind the starting (scratch) line. Bend your knees, and bring your hands below your waist. Then hop as far as you can on one leg, extending fully with your ankles, knees, hips, and arms.

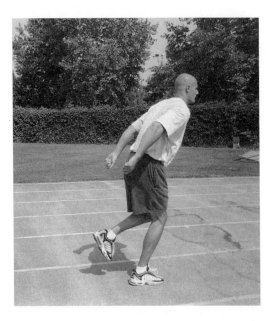

■ **FIGURE 6.13b**

Land on the same leg from which you took off, and then step vigorously with the other leg. As you land, immediately jump with that leg and complete the exercise. In a possible sequence, you might hop with the right leg, extend and land on the left leg (step), and complete the jump with the left leg.

Skiers (Figure 6.14)

Skiers is a good exercise for alpine and cross-country skiers, skaters, and people who must change direction rapidly when running.

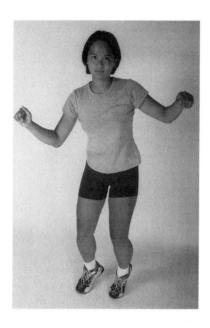

■ FIGURE 6.14a

Stand with your feet together.

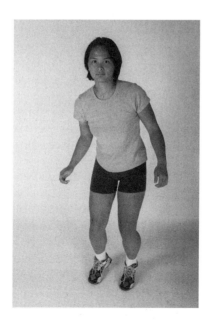

■ FIGURE 6.14b

With both feet still together, jump forward and to the left side, land, and then jump forward and to the right. Jump as quickly as possible for 5–10 repetitions. You have finished one repetition when you have jumped to the left and right sides.

Four Squares (Figure 6.15)

This exercise also builds leg power for lateral movements.

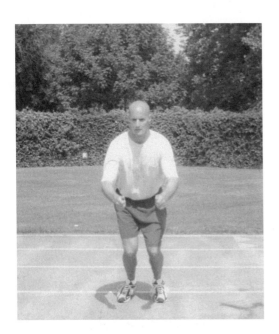

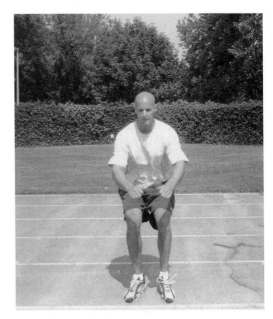

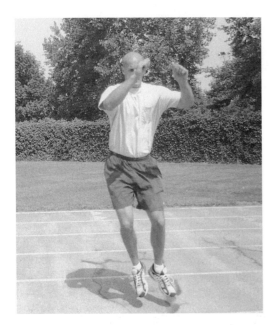

■ **FIGURE 6.15a–c**

Stand with your feet together on the inside of four markers (small cones, shirts, shoes, etc.) placed approximately 5 feet apart. Keeping your feet together, jump in various patterns in the direction of the markers. For example, if the markers are numbered 1, 2, 3, 4; a jumping sequence might be 1, center, 2, center, 3, center, 4, center. Another combination might be center, 1, 2, 4, 3, center. Many combinations are possible.

Cone Hops (Figure 6.16)

Although similar to the multiple standing long jumps, in this exercise you try to jump for height over the cones as well as distance.

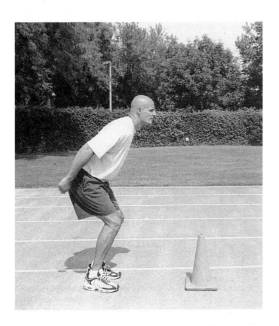
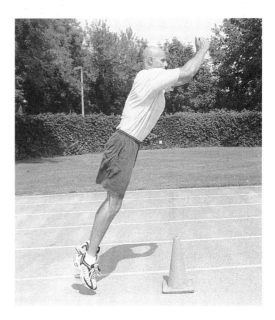
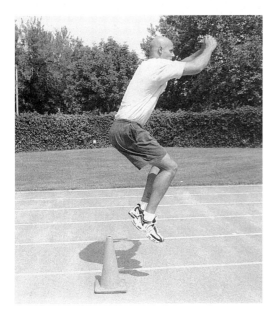

■ **FIGURE 6.16a–c**

Space 3–6 large, 2 foot cones (or similar objects) approximately 3 feet apart. Stand in front of the first cone with your feet shoulder width apart. Jump over the cones as quickly as possible.

Hurdle Hops (Figure 6.17)

This advanced form of cone hops uses hurdles. Do not attempt this exercise unless you are well conditioned and have good jumping ability and technique. If the hurdles have adjustable stabilization weights, make sure they are set so that the hurdle falls down easily if hit. You can construct minihurdles from PVC pipe that are safer for the beginner.

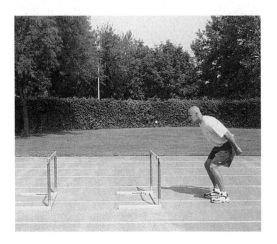 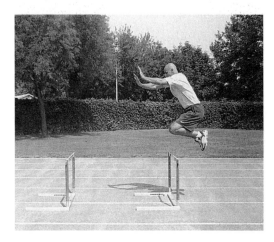

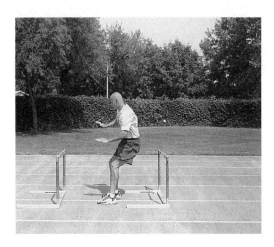

■ **FIGURE 6.17a–c**

Place 3–5 hurdles approximately 3 feet apart. Start with the hurdle at its lowest height. Keeping your feet shoulder width apart, hop over the hurdles as quickly as possible using both legs.

Bounce Push-Ups

You can do bounce push-ups, excellent exercises for developing pushing power in the upper body, against a wall, a steeplechase hurdle, or the floor.

Wall Bounce Push-Ups (Figure 6.18)

These exercises are the simplest, least stressful push-ups. Perform these until your muscles and joints become accustomed to the stress of upper-body plyometric exercise.

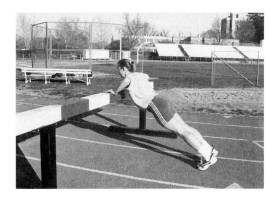

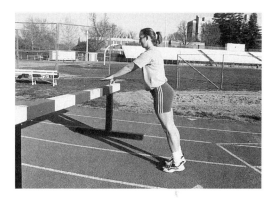

■ **FIGURE 6.18a**

Lean against a wall or steeplechase hurdle at a 45–60° angle.

■ **FIGURE 6.18b**

Push up forcefully; then allow yourself to go back against the wall and to absorb your fall with your arms. Immediately, push off again.

Floor Bounce Push-Ups (Figure 6.19)

These exercises are more stressful and difficult than wall push-ups; do not attempt these until you can do at least 10–15 push-ups. They can be done from a standard or modified push-up position. In the modified push-up position, you rest your weight on your knees instead of your toes.

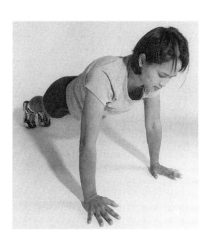

■ **FIGURE 6.19**

From a standard or modified push-up position, push up forcefully, fully extending your elbows until your hands leave the ground. Bounce back to your hands; then repeat the exercise.

Box Jumping

Box jumping requires jumping to and from boxes, benches, or steps. Landing creates more stress on the muscles and joints, so these exercises should be attempted only after doing exercises in which you jump to and from the ground. Box height can vary from approximately 6 inches to 5 feet. Start with smaller boxes, and progress slowly to higher ones. As with other plyometric exercises, the object is to attempt to jump as soon as possible after you land.

Step Downs (Figure 6.20)

This exercise is the simplest, least stressful box jump. You should begin with a low box (approximately 1–2 feet high) and should progress from simply stepping down from the box and absorbing the shock with the legs to jumping down, landing, and vigorously jumping into the air. Finally, you should jump between a series of boxes.

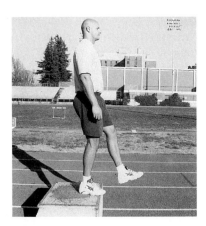

■ FIGURE 6.20a

Phase 1, step downs.
Stand on a box or bench with your feet at shoulder width, knees bent, and spine erect.

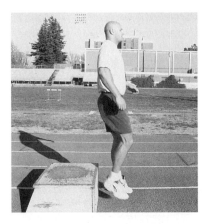

■ FIGURE 6.20b

Step off the bench and land with bent knees.

Phase 2, step down, jump up.   Stand on a box or bench with your feet at shoulder width, knees bent, and spine erect. Step off the bench, land with bent knees, and immediately jump up using both legs and arms.

Phase 3, repeat step down, jump up.   Place 3–6 boxes or benches approximately 3 feet apart. Jump from the first box to the ground, up to the next box, then to the ground, and so forth. Jump as quickly as possible between benches.

Standing Long Jumps from a Box (Figure 6.21)

Although somewhat similar to standing long jumps, this exercise, sometimes called *depth jumping,* stresses your legs more when you land.

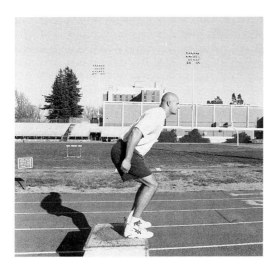

■ **FIGURE 6.21a**

Stand on a box or bench with your feet placed shoulder width apart.

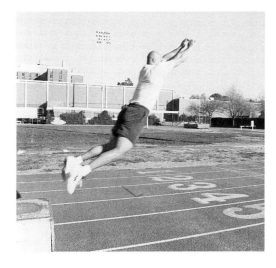

■ **FIGURE 6.21b**

Jump as far as possible, extending fully your ankles, knees, hips, and arms. Land with bent knees. As your fitness improves, increase the height of the box. A variation of this exercise is to land on the ground, and then jump (standing long jump) again immediately.

Ski Box Jumps (Figure 6.22)

Somewhat similar to skiers, in this exercise you jump to and from a box as you jump side-to-side.

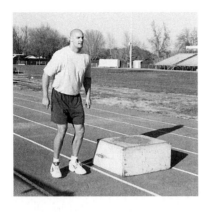

■ FIGURE 6.22a
Stand with your side to a box or bench.

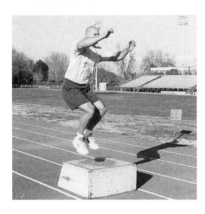

■ FIGURE 6.22b
With your feet together, jump up vigorously onto the bench.

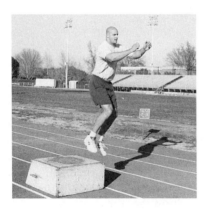

■ FIGURE 6.22c
Immediately jump to the ground on the other side. Then jump back to the bench. Finally, jump back to the starting position.

Single-Leg Jump-Ups (Figure 6.23)

This exercise isolates powerful thigh muscles and develops your jumping power in activities involving a single-leg takeoff (e.g., layup in basketball, jumping for the ball when running).

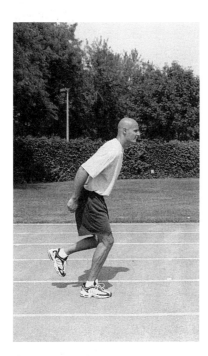 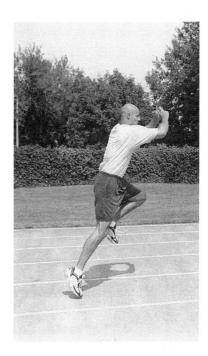

■ FIGURE 6.23a–b

Beginning from the ground, drive hard with your leg, extend fully your ankle, knee, and hip, and jump into the air; land on one leg. Then repeat immediately. As you progress, take off from a box or bench.

Medicine Ball Exercises

A medicine ball resembles a basketball in size but is heavier and softer; it is usually made of leather. However, newer medicine balls are sometimes made of rubber, and some even have handles. Medicine balls weigh from 2 to 20 pounds and, because of their weight, are excellent for plyometrics. When you catch them, your muscles stretch and contract eccentrically as you attempt to slow down and control the ball. You can do medicine ball exercises by yourself or with a partner.

Play Catch with Yourself (Figure 6.24)

Do this exercise with the ball starting from your chest, behind the neck, or at your waist. These activities are good whole-body exercises because you must use your legs, arms, and trunk to perform them properly.

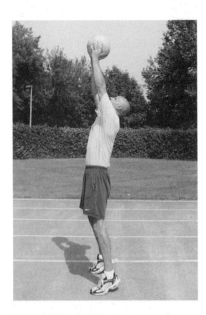

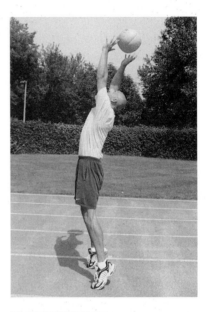

■ **FIGURE 6.24a**

Chest-high catch. Stand with your feet shoulder width apart, and hold the ball with both hands at chest level. Vigorously press the ball overhead with both hands until it flies into the air straight above you; use your legs to help push the ball overhead.

■ **FIGURE 6.24b**

Catch the ball with both hands, and immediately throw the ball into the air again. Repeat.

Behind-the-neck catch. Stand with your feet shoulder width apart, and hold the ball behind your head with both hands. Vigorously press the ball overhead with both hands until it flies into the air straight above you; use your legs to help push the ball overhead. Catch the ball behind your head with both hands, and immediately throw the ball into the air again. Repeat. Do not do this exercise if you have shoulder problems. Start with a light medicine ball (2–5 pounds) before progressing to a heavier one.

Waist-high catch.   Stand with your feet shoulder width apart, and place your hands under the ball at waist level. Vigorously push the ball overhead with both hands until it flies into the air straight above you; use your legs to help push the ball overhead. Catch the ball with both hands, and immediately throw the ball into the air again. Repeat. As you become accustomed to this exercise, jump into the air as you throw the ball, land, catch the ball, and repeat.

Medicine Ball or Shot Put Throws (Figure 6.25)

You can also develop power by throwing a medicine ball or shot put in various ways. Exercises include overhead, underhand, and side-rotation throws.

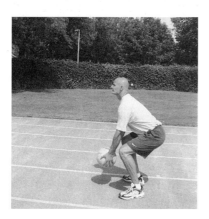
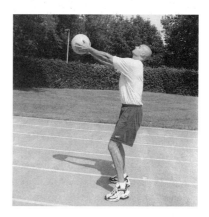

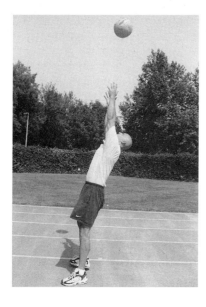

■ **FIGURE 6.25a–c**

Overhead throw.   The motion for this exercise is similar to the underhand throw described on the next page, but you throw the medicine ball or shot put over your head and behind you. Try to throw the object as far overhead as possible. Extend fully the ankles, knees, hips, and arms, and jump from the ground as you throw the ball.

Front waist throw. This underhand throw is initiated at the waist, but you must throw the ball or shot put in front of you. You can also throw the ball from your waist in front of you or rotating to the side.

Waist throw to the side. Hold the ball or shot in both hands. Rotate to the right, and then to the left. Then, throw the object as far as possible. Try to transfer your weight from the rear to the front foot during the throw. Repeat the exercise on the other side of the body.

Medicine Ball Exercises with a Partner

These exercises develop power in the upper and lower body. Variations are limited only by your imagination.

Chest Passes (Figure 6.26)

This exercise develops the pushing muscles in the upper body and strengthens the muscles of the trunk and lower body.

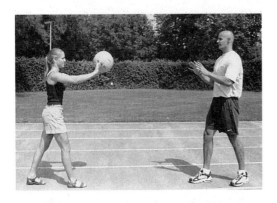

■ **FIGURE 6.26a**

Stand with one foot in front of the other with your knees bent slightly, approximately 6–10 feet from a partner. Hold the ball in both hands at chest level, and throw it to your partner using a motion similar to a basketball chest pass.

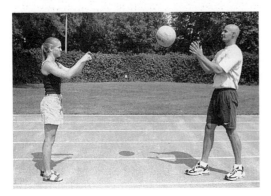

■ **FIGURE 6.26b**

Your partner should catch the ball.

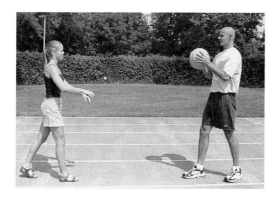

■ **FIGURE 6.26c**

Your partner should immediately throw it back to you; the catching motion should blend continuously with the throwing motion in a semicircular pattern. You can also do this exercise from a kneeling position if you want to isolate the upper-body muscles.

Overhead Passes (Figure 6.27)

This exercise develops power in your triceps and shoulder muscles. Beware of this exercise if you have shoulder problems.

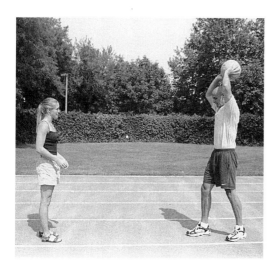

■ **FIGURE 6.27**

Stand facing your partner, approximately 6–10 feet apart. Hold the ball in both hands behind your head. Throw the ball forward over your head so that your partner catches it with arms extended overhead. Your partner then retracts the ball overhead and throws it back to you.

Medicine Ball Sit-Ups (Figure 6.28)

Two athletes can do this together, or you can do this exercise by yourself with a spotter. Do not attempt to do this exercise until you have conditioned your abdominal and back muscles with standard exercises (e.g., sit-ups, crunches, back extensions, etc.).

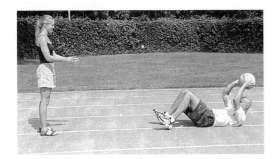

■ **FIGURE 6.28a**

One person with spotter. Although similar to the 2-person sit-ups, in this exercise a spotter or coach stands 3–5 feet from the person doing the sit-ups.

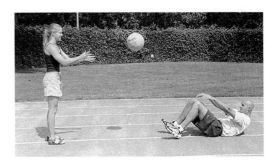

■ **FIGURE 6.28b**

At the top of the sit-up, the person tosses the ball to the spotter and completes a sit-up without the medicine ball.

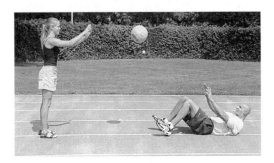

■ **FIGURE 6.28c**

Then, he or she returns to the top of the sit-up.

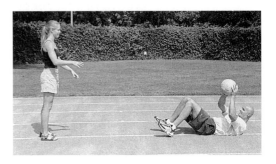

■ **FIGURE 6.28d**

The person catches the ball that the spotter throws. The sequence is as follows: Sit-up with the ball, throw the ball to the spotter, sit-up without the ball, catch the ball from the spotter, and repeat.

Two-person sit-ups. Sit facing each other with your knees bent and your feet flat on the floor; meanwhile, one person holds the medicine ball. Both people should go backward with their hands overhead until their backs reach the ground; then, both sit up at the same time. As the person with the ball reaches the top of the sit-up, he or she tosses the ball to the other person who then catches it. They repeat the exercise, tossing the ball to the other person at the top of each sit-up. The sequence for each person is as follows: Sit-up with the ball, throw the ball to your partner, sit-up without the ball, catch the ball from your partner, and repeat.

Olympic Weight Lifting

Olympic weight lifting is a competitive sport that includes the clean, the jerk, and the snatch exercises. These extremely dynamic lifts work the large muscles of the upper and lower body. Although these lifts do not transfer power immediately to sports skills, they do provide a strength and power base that will eventually help you improve in many strength–speed sports. This chapter will describe the power clean, jerk, and snatch, which are modifications of the exercises done by Olympic weight lifters.

Find a coach to teach you the Olympic lifts. Posture and technique are critical for preventing injury and making satisfactory progress; a good coach will help you avoid common mistakes and progress rapidly in these exciting and beneficial exercises.

Power Clean (Figure 6.29)

This exercise develops power in the muscles used for jumping and pulling objects from the floor; it is a core exercise for strength–speed athletes, such as throwers, football players, volleyball and basketball players.

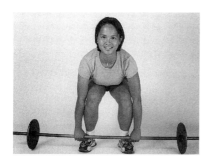

■ **FIGURE 6.29a**

Place the bar on the floor in front of your shins and keep your feet approximately two feet apart. Grasp the bar with your palms facing you and your hands shoulder-width apart.

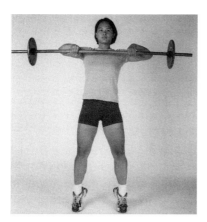

■ **FIGURE 6.29b**

As you squat, keep your arms and back straight and your head up. Pull the weight up past your knees to your chest while throwing your hips forward and your shoulders back.

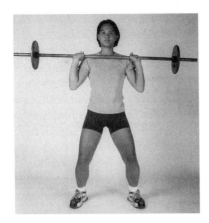

■ **FIGURE 6.29c**

After pulling the weight as high as you can, bend your knees suddenly, and catch the bar on your chest at a level just above your collarbone. Stand up straight with the bar at chest level. Then, return the bar to the starting position. The main power for this exercise should come from your hips and legs. To drive up the weight with your legs rather than your arms, think of the middle phase of the lift as a vertical jump.

Variations: Variations of this lift include the high pull and the squat clean. The high pull is identical to the power clean except that you do not turn the bar over at the top of the lift and catch it at your chest. This procedure allows you to handle more weight and to place less stress on your wrists and forearms.

The squat clean is a technically more difficult lift than the power clean. At the top of the pulling phase of the clean, bend your knees fully, and catch the weight at your chest while in a full squat. When you master this movement, you will be able to clean more weight than you can power clean because you do not have to pull the weight as high.

Power Snatch (Figure 6.30)

The power snatch is more complex and difficult than the power clean. The object of the lift is to pull the bar over your head in one movement and catch it overhead with your arms straight. Good coaching is essential to mastering this lift.

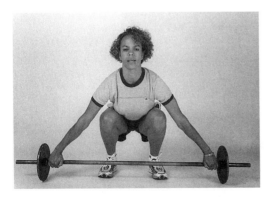

■ **FIGURE 6.30a**

Place the bar on the floor in front of your shins, and keep your feet approximately two feet apart. Grasp the bar with your palms facing you and your hands placed as far apart as possible.

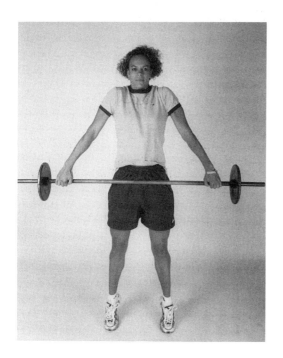

■ **FIGURE 6.30b**

As you squat, keep your arms and back straight and your head up. Pull the weight up past your knees to your chest while throwing your hips forward and your shoulders back.

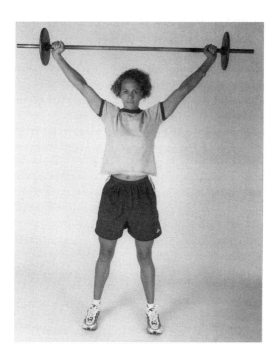

■ **FIGURE 6.30c**

After pulling the weight as high as you can, bend your knees suddenly, and catch it overhead with your arms straight. Stand up straight with the bar overhead. Return the bar to the starting position.

Jerk (Figure 6.31)

To the novice, the jerk looks like a shoulder or military press described in Chapter 4, but the jerk is mainly a leg exercise. You hoist the bar overhead by driving with your legs and dropping underneath the bar.

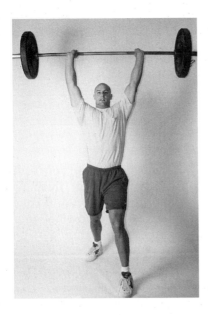

■ **FIGURE 6.31**

Begin this exercise with the bar at the top of the clean position, resting on your chest approximately at the level of your collarbone. You can get the bar to this position by doing a clean or taking the bar from a rack placed at chest level (this exercise is called *jerks off the rack*). Next, bend your knees, and push the bar up vigorously using your legs and arms. Drop underneath the bar using a split movement, one leg forward with bent knee and the other leg extended straight to the back. Finally, bring your feet together so that you are in a standing position with the bar overhead and in control.

Other Exercises to Develop Speed and Power

Chapters 5 and 6 have presented samples of speed and power exercises. Variations are limited only by your imagination. Because you cannot include all the exercises presented in your exercise program, choose those whose movements most closely resemble your favorite sports. In general, choose about 6–12 speed and power exercises, and integrate them into a program that includes cardiovascular, strength, and flexibility exercises. Sample exercise routines and exercise programming are discussed in Chapter 8.

Remember, the power you gain from these exercises will not transfer automatically to increased power in your sport. You must practice the skill and gradually integrate your increased power into your movements. If you work consistently on sports skills and do exercises to increase strength and power, you will eventually become more powerful in your sport.

7

Flexibility

Flexibility, the ability to move a joint through its range of motion, is an extremely important fitness component for health and performance, yet it is perhaps the least studied and most misunderstood area of fitness.

Good flexibility is important for normal joint function and injury prevention. Flexible hip and back joints help maintain proper spinal alignment that prevents back pain; flexible knees, shoulders, and ankles prevent stresses and injuries to their supporting muscle groups and soft tissues. Good flexibility also helps to maintain pain-free joint movement as you get older. There is even some evidence that your ability to increase strength through resistance exercises may be impaired if your flexibility is inadequate. Smooth performance of many movements in sports and daily living are impossible if you have less than normal flexibility.

Joint flexibility is a highly adaptable physical fitness quality that is specific to each joint; if you have good flexibility in one joint, you will not necessarily have good flexibility in another. If you move a joint regularly through its range of motion, that joint will tend to have good flexibility. For example, gymnasts generally have extremely good spinal flexibility, and tennis players tend to have excellent flexibility in their shoulders. Because these athletes stress the affected joints to the limits of their movement capacities, they tend to have excellent flexibility in those joints. The main factor that determines flexibility seems to be the extent to which you stress each joint to the limits of its range of motion.

However, you will lose flexibility if you do not exercise much or move your joints regularly through their normal ranges of motion. Unfit people tend to be less flexible than physically fit people—so much so that joint stiffness can interfere with movements important in everyday life. For example, rising from a chair or reaching overhead for objects stored in a cabinet are more difficult when you have poor flexibility. Deteriorating flexibility will eventually impair normal joint function and become a handicapping condition, so doing exercises that contribute to flexibility (i.e., exercises that work the joints through their normal ranges of motion or specific stretching exercises) is important for general fitness and wellness.

What Determines Flexibility?

Your ability to move a joint is limited by tissues that prevent movement (i.e., the tissues either get in the way of movement or provide resistance to further movement) and muscle length set by the nervous system. Although some of these factors, such as bone structure, cannot change, others, such as the resting length of elastic soft tissues, can be altered through exercise.

Tissues That Obstruct Range of Motion

Bones limit movement in many joints—the structure of the bones forming many joints allows joint movement to proceed only so far. These *bony stops* give strength and stability to joints, making them important to human movement. Surrounding the major joints of the body are joint capsules, which are semielastic structures that limit movement and give joints strength and stability. While they can be stretched slightly, they are semirigid and resist deformation.

The body contains numerous soft tissues that can limit flexibility; fat, skin, and large muscles can get in the way and prevent a joint from moving through a larger range of motion. For example, people with extremely large biceps cannot fully flex (bend) their elbows because the upper muscle gets in the way. Obese people cannot make certain movements, such as flexing the trunk completely, because excess body fat impedes the range of motion. Extremely tight skin, stretched by large muscles, body fat, or pregnancy, can also interfere with movement.

Muscle Elasticity

Muscle tissue is the key to developing flexibility. In addition to the contractile proteins that create movement within muscles, muscles contain collagenous tissues that provide structure, elasticity, and bulk to the muscle. The two principle types of collagenous tissues are collagen, white fibers that provide structure and support, and elastin, yellow fibers that are elastic and flexible. The elastin fibers have the capacity to be stretched and rapidly snapped back to their resting position when the stretch is relieved. If the fibers are loaded at low levels of stress (e.g., during exercises that gently stress the joints to the limits of their ranges of motion), then the elastin fibers get longer; in other words, they stretch.

Of course, there is a limit to the amount of stretch a muscle will tolerate. If stretched too much, the collagen will not return to its resting shape, and an injury results. Collagen increases in stiffness as it is stretched; as the limits of its flexibility are reached, the collagen becomes more brittle and may rupture if overstretched. The stretch characteristics of elastin tissue in muscle are important considerations in a stretching program. You must stretch the muscle enough to lengthen the elastin tissue, but if you overstretch a muscle, you may cause serious injury. The effects of stretch on elastin tissue is shown in Figure 7.1. The effective and safe stretching program is one that stresses the muscle enough to slightly elongate and stretch the elastin fibers, but not so much that they cannot return to their normal shape.

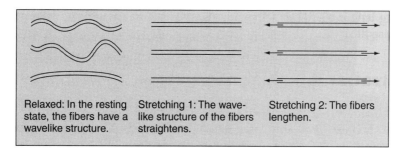

Relaxed: In the resting state, the fibers have a wavelike structure.

Stretching 1: The wave-like structure of the fibers straightens.

Stretching 2: The fibers lengthen.

FIGURE 7.1   The Effects of Stretch on Elastin Tissue.

Nervous System Control of Muscle Length

Muscles contain stretch receptors that control the muscles' lengths. If a muscle is stretched suddenly, stretch receptors send signals to the spinal cord that in turn sends a signal back to the muscle, causing it to contract. These reflexes occur frequently in active muscle and are important for control of movement. They help the body know what the muscles are doing and allow for control of muscle length. Small movements that stimulate the receptors result in small reflex activity from the spinal cord.

Rapid, powerful, and sudden movements that greatly stretch the receptors result in large, powerful reflex muscle contractions. Ballistic stretching, stretching involving rapid, bouncy movements, is considered dangerous because it may stimulate a reflex muscle contraction during the exercise. In other words, the muscle may be contracting while it is being stretched, causing it to become injured easily. For that reason, you should stretch statically—stretch the muscle and hold the stretch.

Strong muscle contractions also induce a neural reflex that causes muscles to relax. Muscle contractions stimulate receptors in muscle tendons called *Golgi tendon organs,* which help to prevent muscles from contracting too hard. The Golgi tendon reflex (sometimes called the *inverse stretch reflex*) has recently been introduced as an aid to improving flexibility. By contracting a muscle prior to stretching it, the muscle relaxes and may allow you to stretch it more than normal. The contraction–stretch technique for developing flexibility is called *proprioceptive neuromuscular facilitation* (PNF). Recent studies, however, have shown that PNF techniques may not relax muscles as much as previously thought (Knapik et al., 1992).

CHANGING STRETCH RECEPTOR SENSITIVITY.   You can reset the sensitivity of muscle stretch receptors by repeating stretching exercises several times in succession. If you statically stretch a muscle, relax, and then stretch it again, the stretch receptors will become slightly less sensitive and allow you to stretch the muscle further.

Scientists do not know if stretch receptor sensitivity changes after weeks and months of training. They only know that flexibility increases by elongating the

ıgth of muscle connective tissue and that neural changes also help you
exibility.

ching Techniques

Stretching techniques vary from simple stretches during the course of normal activities to sophisticated stretching techniques that use muscle reflexes to get more
stretch during the exercise. Certainly, improper stretching techniques do more harm
than good.

Static Stretching

In static stretching, you stretch the muscle slowly and hold the stretch for 10–30 seconds. Because the stretch occurs slowly, the stetch receptors react less. Static stretching is most recommended by fitness experts because it is effective and safer than
other stretching exercises. The key to this technique is to stretch the muscles and
joints to the point at which you feel a pull, not pain. Overstretching the muscle leads
to injury.

Ballistic Stretching

Ballistic stretching involves dynamic muscle action in which the muscles are
stretched suddenly in a bouncing movement. For example, a ballistic stretch for the
hamstrings might involve touching your toes repeatedly in rapid succession. Unfortunately, rapid stretches invoke a powerful stretch receptor response that can result in injury.

Passive Stretching

In passive stretching, a partner assists you in moving joints through their ranges of
motion. Although you can achieve a greater range of motion passively than you can
statically, because you are not controlling the movement, there is a greater risk of
injury. Passive stretching is a valuable technique that should be used only by experienced people who thoroughly understand the technique. In addition, good communication between the people performing and receiving passive stretches must be
maintained.

Proprioceptive Neuromuscular Facilitation (PNF)

PNF techniques improve strength and flexibility, and they attempt to use reflexes
initiated by muscle and joint receptors to cause greater training effects. The most
popular PNF stretching technique is the contract–relax stretching method—the
muscle is actively contracted before it is stretched. Although some believe that contracting the muscle first causes it to relax more so that it can be stretched more

effectively, the technique is still controversial. Currently, there is no evidence to show that it is any more effective than static stretching (Knapik et al., 1992).

Benefits of Flexibility and Stretching Exercises

Flexibility has wide-ranging benefits for wellness and sports performance. Good flexibility may help prevent injury, enhance joint function, and make movements in many sports easier and more efficient.

Flexibility and Injury

Muscles are injured when they are loaded more than they can tolerate. Muscles can stretch to a point, but if they are stretched too far, then injury results. The flexible joint can move further in the range of motion before reaching critical stresses that cause injury.

Most experts recommend that you stretch before you exercise (Knapik et al., 1992). However, it has not been proven conclusively that pre-exercise stretching prevents injury. In fact, some studies show that stretching before exercise may actually increase the risk of injury, but these findings may be due to improper stretching techniques. Bounce-type ballistic stretching before exercise may increase the activity of muscle stretch receptors leading to an increased chance that the muscle will contract while in a stretched position (a scenario that may result in injury). Static stretching (see below), on the other hand, appears to increase joint range of motion without increasing stretch receptor sensitivity.

Flexibility and Joint Health

Researchers and physicians are becoming increasingly aware that good flexibility is important to good joint health; joints supported by inflexible muscles and soft tissues are subjected to abnormal stresses that can result in joint deterioration (ACSM, 1998). In the knee joint, for example, tight quadriceps and hamstrings cause excessive pressure on the kneecap that can cause pain in the knee joint. Tense shoulder muscles can compress sensitive soft tissues in the shoulder and cause pain and disability in the joint. Poor joint flexibility can also result in abnormalities in joint lubrication that can cause deterioration in the sensitive cartilage cells lining the joint.

Joint Flexibility and Spinal Alignment

Back pain affects nearly 85 percent of the population at some time in their lives. Often, back pain may be related to poor spinal alignment that puts pressure on the nerves emanating from the spinal column. Poor flexibility in the spine, pelvis, and knees can increase the curve of the lower spine and cause the pelvis to tilt forward excessively. Good flexibility in these areas, along with good posture, helps prevent abnormal pressures on sensitive spinal nerves.

Stretching and Postexercise Muscle Soreness

Delayed onset muscle soreness (DOMS), sore muscles occurring one to two days after exercise, is thought to be caused by damage to the muscle fibers and supporting connective tissue. Some, but not all, studies have shown that stretching after exercise decreases muscle soreness after exercise, but scientists cannot explain why postexercise stretching helps to relieve the pain of DOMS (Armstrong et al., 1991). It may decrease muscle spasms that may occur in reaction to the soreness.

Flexibility and Body Position in Sports

Good flexibility lets you move and exert force through a greater range of motion. Flexible people can assume body positions that allow them to move more efficiently. For example, skiers with flexible hips and spines are better able to get over the edge of their skis so that they can turn. Swimmers with more flexible shoulders have a stronger stroke because they can pull through the water in a direction closer to the midline of the body. Hikers with flexible calves and Achilles tendons can climb big hills without pain because of their greater ranges of motion in the lower leg.

Flexibility and Strength

Many people think that weight lifting makes you muscle bound. A look at many weight lifters seems to reinforce this impression—many have large, bulky muscles, and their skins have stretch marks from trying to accommodate the tremendous bulk. Despite their appearances, strong people can also be flexible. In the 1950s, Olympic weight lifter and bodybuilder John Grimek was famous for his displays of flexibility in addition to his great strength. Many great strength athletes of today are also flexible because they work on it.

Scientists have discovered a link between flexibility and strength; they believe that a minimum amount of flexibility is important if you are to gain strength normally. If your flexibility is extremely poor, then you will not gain strength as fast as you would if you had normal flexibility. Research has shown that lack of flexibility in antagonistic muscles may impede the development of muscle strength and hypertrophy (i.e., getting larger muscles) (Knapik et al., 1992). An antagonistic muscle opposes the action of another muscle. For example, the hamstring muscles are the antagonistic muscle group to the quadriceps.

Lack of flexibility in the hamstrings affects the strength of the quadriceps because of the principle of *reciprocal inhibition*. Reciprocal inhibition is the process by which stimulation of the muscle spindles of the antagonist muscle (e.g., the hamstrings) inhibits excitation of the agonist muscle (e.g., the quadriceps) through a neural process involving the spinal cord. The muscle spindles are receptors within the muscles that are sensitive to stretch. In a squat, for example, if the muscle spindles in the hamstrings are stimulated during the pushing phase of the lift, the quadriceps will be inhibited. This inhibition will prevent you from exerting full force during the squat and will keep you from getting stronger in the lift.

Many studies have examined the influence of reciprocal inhibition in limb movement. For example, in the knee-jerk reflex, tapping the patellar tendon produces a stretch reflex by the muscle spindles in the quadriceps muscles that results in contraction of the quadriceps, inhibition of the hamstring muscles, and extension of the knee.

According to this principle, inflexible hamstring muscles may make it more difficult to strengthen knee extensors. During knee extension, premature stimulation of the muscle spindles in the hamstrings could result in reflex inhibition of the quadriceps. Research has shown that quadriceps strength tends to be less in people who have less flexible hamstrings probably because the muscle spindles in the hamstrings turn off the quadriceps during the final phase of most lower-body exercises (Alter, 1988). Chronic quadriceps inhibition keeps these people from getting as strong as they would if they had normal hamstring flexibility.

A minimum amount of flexibility in major muscles seems to be necessary to prevent strength impairment in the antagonistic muscles. For example, when hamstring flexibility is less than the flexibility threshold, a significant portion of its muscle spindle may be prematurely stimulated during knee extension, resulting in a premature stretch reflex response in the hamstrings and a reflex inhibition of the knee extensors.

Do these findings mean you should spend 4–5 hours a week stretching? No, flexibility will only impair strength if you are extremely tight. Research does not suggest that if you become extremely flexible, you will improve strength at a faster rate. It shows that if you are inflexible, your progress will be impeded (Alter, 1988). For an extremely inflexible person, working on flexibility may make it easier to gain strength. Presently, the examination of strength and flexibility has been limited to the relationship between hamstring flexibility and quadriceps strength. However, there is no reason to think that the muscle spindles work differently in areas other than the legs.

Several studies suggest that stretching before exercise might decrease performance in maximum power exercises, such as jumping and throwing (Alter, 1988). As discussed, stretching stimulates the golgi tendon organs that act to limit muscle tension. After you stretch, if you try to exert maximum power or strength, the golgi tendon organs will be stimulated and will hamper performance. It is better to warm up by doing low-intensity dynamic exercises. Because stretching before exercise may lead to injury and decreased performance, it will remain controversial for many years to come.

Principles of Flexibility

Ideally, do stretching exercises after you exercise. If you stretch as part of the warm-up, perform general, low-intensity warm-up exercises before stretching. The muscles will be warmer, and there will be less risk of injury. To greatly improve flexibility, stretch after you exercise because the muscles are warmer and will stretch further. The following principles should also be followed as part of your stretching program.

- Do stretching exercises statically. Stretch and hold the position for 10–30 seconds, rest 30–60 seconds, and repeat. Never bounce while stretching because it increases the risk of injury.
- Practice stretching exercises regularly, and develop flexibility gradually over time. Improved flexibility, like other types of fitness, takes many months to develop.
- Do gentle warm-up exercises, such as easy jogging or calisthenics, before doing your pre-exercise stretching routine.
- Note that you should feel a mild stretch rather than pain while performing these exercises. Emphasize relaxation.
- Do all flexibility exercises on both sides of the body.
- Avoid positions that increase the risk of lower back injury. For example, if you are performing straight-leg, toe-touching exercises, bend your knees slightly when returning to a standing position.
- Note that there are large individual differences in joint flexibility. Do not feel you must compete with others during stretching workouts.

Basic Stretching Exercises and Your Stretching Routine

Whole Body Stretches

- "Good-Morning" Stretch
- "Good-Morning" Stretch with Toe Touches

Lower Body Stretches

- Supine Alternate Hamstring Stretch
- Modified Hurdler Stretch
- Standing Calf Stretch
- Lunge Stretch
- Groin Stretch

Trunk and Back Stretches

- Standing Side Stretch
- Trunk Rotation Stretch
- Pelvic Tilt
- Supine Trunk Twist

Shoulder and Upper Torso Exercises

- Across-the-Body Shoulder Stretch
- Chest Stretch

Literally hundreds of possible stretching exercises exist. Choose exercises that stretch the major muscle groups in the body. Try to stretch a little every day, or at least 5 days per week. Choose a regular stretching time; a good choice is in the morning right after you wake up or in the evening prior to going to bed. Do not try to become flexible in one day. Build up stretching intensity gradually.

Whole Body Stretches

"Good-Morning" Stretch (Figure 7.2)

This simple stretch is particularly good to do after you wake up in the morning. This exercise helps to stretch your spine and shoulders.

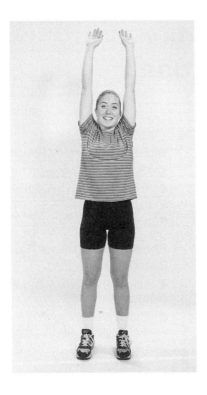

■ **FIGURE 7.2**

Stand with your feet shoulder width apart, and reach up over your head with your arms extended fully. Try to extend your arms as much as possible—first one arm, then the other, then both arms. Hold each stretch for at least 10 seconds.

"Good-Morning" Stretch with Toe Touches (Figure 7.3)

Although similar to the last exercise, in this exercise you add toe touches to the stretching sequence.

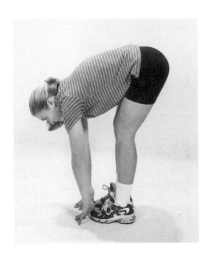

■ **FIGURE 7.3**

Stand with your feet shoulder width apart, and reach up over your head with your arms extended fully. Try to extend your arms as much as possible—first one arm, then the other, then both arms. Then, flex your knees slightly, bend over at the waist, and reach toward your toes. Reach down until you feel the stretch in your hamstring muscles. Hold the stretch for 10–30 seconds. Repeat the total exercise.

Lower Body Stretches

Supine Alternate Hamstring Stretch (Figure 7.4)

This excellent exercise stretches your back, hamstrings, hips, knees, ankles, and buttocks.

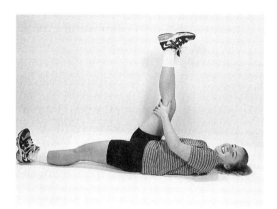

■ **FIGURE 7.4**

Lie on your back with both legs straight. Grasp the back of your right thigh, and bring your knee to your chest (this segment is sometimes called the *knee-to-chest exercise*). Pull on your thigh until you feel a stretch in your lower back. Hold the stretch for 10–30 seconds. Then, extend your knee so that you feel a stretch in the back of your right hamstring muscles (*supine hamstring stretch*). Hold the stretch, and return to the starting position. You can also do knee-to-chest and supine hamstring stretches separately.

Modified Hurdler Stretch (Figure 7.5)

This exercise stretches the hamstring muscles and lower back. Avoid doing hurdler stretches in which you sit with one leg stretched out to the side as you stretch the other extended leg. Turning out the bent leg can put excessive strain on the ligaments of the knee.

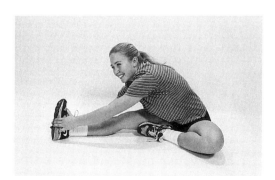

■ **FIGURE 7.5**

Sit with your right leg straight and your left leg tucked close to your body. Reach as far as possible toward your right foot. Repeat for the other leg.

Standing Calf Stretch (Figure 7.6)

Flexible calf muscles help to prevent knee, ankle, and foot pain. This exercise helps to stretch the calf muscles (gastrocnemius and soleus) and the Achilles tendon.

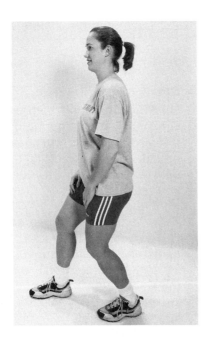

■ **FIGURE 7.6**

This is a two-part exercise (a and b). Stand with one foot about 1–2 feet in front of the other, with both feet pointing forward. (a) Keeping your back leg straight, lunge forward by bending your front knee and pushing your rear heel backward. Hold the stretch for 10–30 seconds. (b) Then, pull your back foot in slightly, and bend your back knee. Shift your weight to your back leg, and hold the stretch. Repeat this exercise on the other side.

Lunge Stretch (Figure 7.7)

This exercise stretches the hip, thigh, and calf muscles.

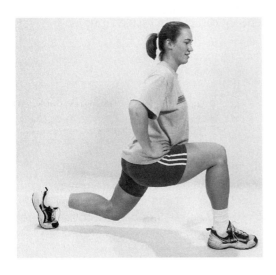

■ **FIGURE 7.7**

Step forward in a lunge with your right foot, and flex your knee. Keep your knee directly above your ankle. Then, stretch your left leg back so that it is parallel to the floor, and press your hips forward and down until you feel a stretch in your quadriceps muscles. Hold the stretch. Balance yourself by placing your arms at your sides, on the top of your knee, or on the ground. Repeat the exercise on your left side.

Groin Stretch (Figure 7.8)

The groin muscles attach to the inside portion of your pelvis and are extremely important for lateral movements. These muscles are injured often in strength–speed sports that require you to sprint and change directions quickly (e.g., tennis, basketball, soccer, racquetball, field hockey).

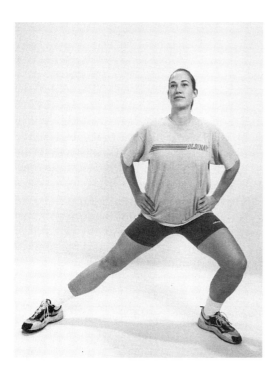

■ **FIGURE 7.8**

Stand in a wide straddle with your legs turned out from your hip joints and your hands on your thighs. Go to one side by bending one knee and keeping the other leg straight. You should feel a stretch in the muscles on the inside of your thigh of the extended leg. Repeat on the other side.

Trunk and Back Stretches

Trunk and back flexibility is essential to fluid movement and a pain-free back. An excellent exercise that stretches the lower back muscles and the power hip flexors (iliopsoas muscle group) is the knee-to-chest exercise, which has already been described (see Figure 7.4).

Standing Side Stretch (Figure 7.9)

This exercise stretches many muscles in your trunk, particularly the obliques.

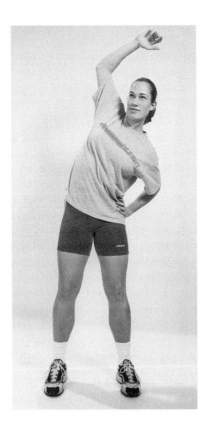

■ **FIGURE 7.9**

Stand with your feet shoulder width apart, knees slightly bent, and pelvis tucked under. Raise one arm over your head, and bend sideways from the waist. Support your trunk by placing the hand or forearm of your other arm on your thigh or hip. Be sure to bend directly sideways, and do not move your body below the waist. Repeat on the other side.

Trunk Rotation Stretch (Figure 7.10)

This stretch is great for the trunk, outer thigh and hip, and lower back.

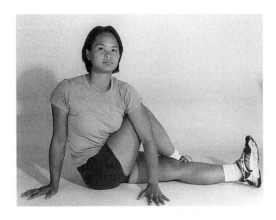

■ **FIGURE 7.10**

Sit with your left leg straight, right leg bent and crossed over the left knee, and right hand on the floor next to your right hip. Turn your trunk as far as possible to the right by pushing against your right leg with your left forearm or elbow. Keep your right foot on the floor. Repeat on the other side.

Pelvic Tilt (Figure 7.11)

This exercise stretches the hip and back muscles and helps to prevent excessive curvature of the lower back.

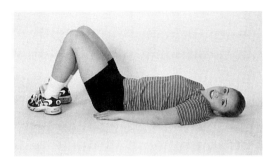

■ **FIGURE 7.11**

Lie on your back with your knees bent and your arms extended to the side. Tilt your pelvis under, and try to flatten your lower back against the floor. Tighten your buttock and abdominal muscles while you hold this position for 5–10 seconds. Do not hold your breath. You can also do this exercise while standing or leaning against a wall.

Supine Trunk Twist (Figure 7.12)

This exercise develops spine and hip flexibility and is also helpful for many people who have back pain.

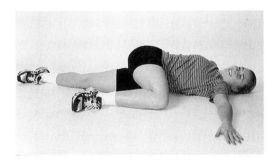

■ **FIGURE 7.12**

Lie on your side with your top knee bent, lower leg straight, lower arm extended out in front of you on the floor, and upper arm at your side. Push down with your upper knee while you twist your trunk backward. Try to get your shoulders and upper body flat on the floor, turning your head as well. Return to the starting position, and repeat on the other side.

Shoulder and Upper Torso Exercises

Because the shoulder is the most mobile joint in the body, there are many different shoulder stretches. This chapter will only present two—one for the muscles of the shoulder and upper back and one for the shoulder and chest.

Across-the-Body Shoulder Stretch (Figure 7.13)

This exercise stretches the shoulder and upper back. To increase the stretch, you can also do it with a partner.

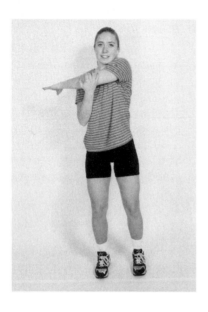

■ **FIGURE 7.13**

From a standing position, cross your left arm in front of your body, and grasp it with your right hand. Stretch your arm, shoulders, and back by gently pulling your arm as close to your body as possible. Repeat the stretch with your right arm.

Chest Stretch (Figure 7.14)

This exercise stretches the muscles of your chest and shoulders.

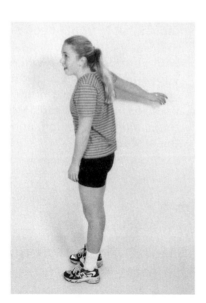

■ **FIGURE 7.14**

Stand to the side of a wall or post at approximately 2–3 feet away. Place your arm on the wall at shoulder level, and walk forward until you feel a stretch in your chest and shoulder muscles. Hold the stretch. Then repeat using the other side of your body.

Other Stretching Exercises

As discussed, there are countless stretching exercises. If you have injuries, such as tennis elbow or shin splints, you may need to do special exercises to help rehabilitate those parts of the body. Consult a physical therapist, athletic trainer, or exercise physiologist for stretching exercises that might be appropriate for your special needs.

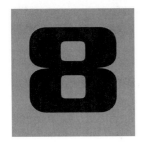

Designing Your Exercise Program

Planning an effective exercise training program is as much art as it is science. You have to consider your goals, strengths and weaknesses, likes and dislikes, and motivation. Equipment and facilities are important—you will not be able to swim if you do not have access to a pool or do Olympic weight lifts if you cannot use free weights. When you design a program, consider what is possible and what exercises you will actually do. A scientifically sophisticated training program is worthless if you never go to the gym.

You can make gains on almost any training program if you stick with it. Plan a realistic program, and do it consistently. Do not search for the single, correct training program because it does not exist. Learn all you can about training, and seek the advice of a good coach, trainer, or exercise physiologist. Try your new program, evaluate it, and then modify it. Soon, you will have a program that works for you.

You should begin conservatively. When you can complete a minimal program, add exercises or train more intensely. Consistency is the key. Follow the principles of training in Table 8.1, and you will likely achieve your goal with a minimum risk of injury.

TABLE 8.1 Principles of Training

Train specifically	Cycle the volume and intensity of your workouts
Establish realistic goals	
Have a workout plan	Work on your weaknesses
Condition your body gradually	Eat a healthy diet
Train consistently	Train your mind
Train first for volume and only later for intensity	Learn all you can about your sport
	Have fun!
Do not overtrain	

Principles of Training

As discussed throughout the book, the purpose of exercise training is to coax your body into adapting to an exercise stress. The stress must be severe enough to stimulate an adaptation but not so severe that you get injured or overtrained. You improve fitness and sports skills by making a series of small adaptations.

The principles of training, shown in Table 8.1, are applicable to anyone who wants to be physically fit. Use these principles even if you simply want to get in great shape.

Train Specifically

The most important training principle to remember is that your body adapts to stress in a specific way. For example, if you swim, you will not improve endurance for running or cycling. Likewise, if you lift weights, you will not become a better football player, discus thrower, skier, or swimmer unless you practice the sport. The best way to improve performance in a sport is to practice that particular sport.

Doing support exercises for your sport, such as weight training, power exercises, and endurance training, will *eventually* improve performance. However, improvement occurs only if you practice the skill and incorporate your new fitness (i.e., strength, power, flexibility, endurance) into it.

Improved fitness can sometimes temporarily decrease performance because your nervous system needs time to precisely program sports skills. When you increase strength, power, flexibility, or endurance in a short time, your brain needs time to adjust to your new capabilities. In the long run, your new fitness will improve your performance. However, this improvement will occur only if your nervous system can incorporate your new fitness into the skill.

The principle of specificity should be the central consideration in any training program designed to improve skilled performance. Skill practice in tennis, skiing, discus throwing, football, and softball should be a central part of the program. Support activities designed to improve physical capabilities, such as strength, power, and endurance, are secondary to skill development.

Physical-support activities (e.g., strength and power training) must be consistent and long term. In other words, lifting weights for 2 months before football or track season is practically worthless because the increased strength will not transfer that rapidly to your motor skills. On the other hand, a support program that develops high levels of fitness over a long period of time can be more effectively integrated into your sport. This program will inject greater strength, power, endurance, and flexibility into your movement skills, and you will perform better.

Summarizing this critical principle of specificity—train the way you want your body to adapt. Support activities designed to make you more powerful during sports movements create change slowly. If you develop strength, power, endurance, and flexibility slowly and consistently, you can integrate your new fitness into your sports skills. Improving fitness without practicing the skill will have no effects on your sports performance.

Establish Realistic Goals

Improved fitness occurs when you stress the body and it adapts. Because of the specificity of training, attaining your goals will reflect the nature of the exercise stress (training program). Therefore, your goals should reflect your capability and motivation. Do not try to be an Olympic discus thrower if you are short and gain strength slowly. But, if you are willing to run the necessary mileage to train for a marathon, go ahead and do it. Otherwise, set more modest goals for yourself.

The best advice is to set achievable, short-term goals. A beginning tennis player might set a goal of keeping a rally going for ten strokes, and a beginning golfer might set a short-term goal of putting the ball on the green in two strokes on 25 percent of the holes. A more accomplished athlete, however, may set more difficult goals ranging from running a 6-minute mile to making the Olympic team. The principle is the same for everyone—set goals you can achieve. After you achieve them, reevaluate your program and set new goals. Your new goal might be to maintain your present level, or it could be to achieve a higher level of performance.

Have a Workout Plan

Write down your goals and your methods for achieving them. Do not simply hope that you will look good in a bathing suit next summer. Also, write down a program for achieving your goals. For example, if you want to lose 20 pounds of body fat and increase your muscle mass, set up a realistic program for achieving your goal; a sensible approach might be to lose 1 pound per week and to go to the gym 3 times per week. In addition, you might achieve your goal by minimizing the amount of desserts and fats in your diet and devoting 30–60 minutes a day to aerobic exercise and weight training.

Contrast this method to a more casual approach. It is January, and you are tired of looking bad in your swimsuit during the summer. You want to lose 20 pounds of fat, but you have no plan. From time to time, you exercise and diet but make no progress because you are inconsistent. Soon, it is May, and you have made no progress. You go on a crash weight-loss program and exercise regime. In spite of great pain and suffering, you fail to meet your goal and end up wearing a baggy T-shirt to the beach.

To set up a good workout plan, analyze the elements necessary for achieving your goal. For example, if you want to be a better skier, you must practice skiing and develop good endurance, strength, power, and flexibility. During the off-season, you would systematically improve your physical fitness. Then, once the ski season approaches, shift your emphasis to skill development, and try to maintain fitness.

The football player should follow a similar procedure. After the football season ends, begin a program designed to gain muscle mass and to improve power output capacity. The weight training program should stress the major muscles of your body as well. In addition, do flexibility and endurance exercises to improve overall fitness. In the spring, integrate more power training, such as plyometrics and speed exercises, into the program. During the summer, shift your training emphasis to maintaining strength and maximizing power, speed, and skill.

Contrast this systematic approach with the more common, crash weight training program started two months before the football season. The athlete might gain strength, but there is little improvement in power, speed, or football skills. The athlete wasted the two critical months before the season doing exercises that should have been done during the winter.

Keep a training diary; this is the best way to ensure a systematic program. Write down your program for the next 4 to 6 weeks, and follow your progress in your training diary. Your diary does not have to be fancy; go to the stationary store, and buy a small spiral notebook. Put it in your gym bag, and carry it with you to all your workouts. Record your weight, your feelings each day, your exercises (sets, reps, etc.), your morning heart rate, and your performances (scores of tennis matches, times of intervals, vertical jump distances, etc.). Furthermore, use your training diary to write down tentative workouts for the next 6 weeks. You should even write down a rough workout plan for the next year. Writing down your plan in the training diary will help you get where you want next month and next year.

The training diary helps you maintain consistency in your workouts and is essential to anyone serious about fitness—regardless of whether you are a serious athlete or a person who wants to get in good shape. Start your training diary today!

Condition Your Body Gradually

Fitness is a gradual process of adaptation. If you try to increase your fitness too quickly, you will either get injured or overtrained. High levels of fitness represent many small adaptations. Introducing the stresses of exercise gradually will eventually lead to better fitness with a minimum risk of injury.

Many sports employ crash exercise programs known as "hell-week" and "double days" even though research studies are unanimous in showing that these programs are ineffective, cause unnecessary fatigue, and lead to injury (Neiman, 1999). You cannot force your body to get fit overnight. Attempts to do so almost always backfire and lead to injury and depressed immune function (overtraining makes it difficult for your body to fight disease). Instead of reaching high levels of fitness, athletes must try to play with a cold or flu and muscles so sore that they have trouble moving effectively. Contrast these results with a one-year program that gradually develops fitness. These physically fit people are capable of high levels of injury-free performance because they have conditioned themselves gradually.

Train Consistently

When you miss workouts, you do not improve fitness; you lose the gains you made. Plan a regular time for your exercise program, and stick to it. Do not let things interfere with your workout. All of us have many responsibilities that compete for our time; if fitness and performance are important to you, you must make your workouts a priority. Workouts are your time, so do not let people take this important time away from you.

Train First for Volume and Only Later for Intensity

This principle seems to be at odds with the principle of specificity. You might ask, as a tennis player or skier, why you would want to develop aerobic capacity and muscle endurance if power output and speed are the most important fitness components. The answer is that low-intensity, repetitive exercise prepares your body to withstand more intensive training with less risk of injury.

High-intensity training, designed to develop power and speed, pushes your body to its limit. If you first develop a fitness base and increase the intensity of training gradually, you will develop power and speed with less risk of strains, sprains, and muscle cramps.

Do Not Overtrain

Overtraining is an imbalance between training and recovery. Among many active people, the motto has often been "no pain, no gain." Although you have to work hard to achieve high levels of fitness, too much or too intense training is counterproductive.

Effective training occurs only if your body adapts to the stress of exercise. This adaptation occurs *after exercise.* If you do not give your body a chance to adapt, you will not get stronger and faster, and you will not improve your endurance. Rather, fitness development comes to a halt, and you get injured or sick.

Proper rest is as important as intense training for improving fitness. When you work out, you are trying to get your body to adapt and improve its function. Before every workout, ask yourself, "What is the purpose of this exercise session, and how will it cause my body to adapt?" If you are exhausted or ill, the workout may cause you to lose ground. You are better off resting for a day or two. When you come back, you will be ready for an intense workout that will improve your fitness.

Exercise training is not an exact science. Sometimes you feel great and can train more intensely than planned. Other times, you feel tired and sluggish. Training intensely in this condition will actually impede progress.

Do not use this principle as an excuse to skip workouts. If you listen to your body and it always tells you to rest, you will never improve fitness. Follow a systematic program, but be flexible enough to change it slightly according to how you feel.

Cycle the Volume and Intensity of Your Workouts

Fitness components, such as speed and power, improve best with intense training; however, it is extremely difficult to recover from too many of these difficult workouts. You must balance rest and moderate-intensity workouts with high-intensity exercise sessions.

If you design your program properly, you can actually plan for effective, intense workout sessions. This process requires a lot of trial and error. For example, you might balance an intense interval training session with a day of rest, followed by a more moderate interval training workout. When you do your next intense interval training workout, you will be recovered enough to train at 100 percent.

The same principle applies to weight training. Do not exercise at maximum intensity every time you go into the gym. Most people cannot do maximum large muscle exercises, such as squats, cleans, and bench presses, every workout. Each workout, emphasize one or two exercises. One time, train intensely on the squat; next time, emphasize the bench press or clean.

You do not need to do the same exercises every workout. For developing maximum strength and power, do shoulder press exercises, such as the bench press, and pulling exercises, such as cleans and snatches, 2 times per week. Do squats 3 times in 2 weeks. For each exercise, alternate between intense and moderate workouts. This method will ensure the proper balance between intense and moderate workouts and rest.

Cycle interval training workouts. Practice interval training 2–3 times per week. On interval training days, do shorter, more intense workouts on some days, and longer, less intense intervals on other days. Between interval training workouts, do overdistance workouts (longer distances at a slower pace) or rest. When you do interval training workouts, make sure to rest completely (no exercise) 1–2 days per week.

Work on Your Weaknesses

The inscription etched in marble on the facades of many U.S. libraries (and the temple of Apollo at the Oracle at Delphi), "Know thyself," should probably be put over the local gym, too. You should analyze your weaknesses and correct them systematically. You can do this only if you establish goals and systematically assess your capability of achieving them.

You do not need a degree in exercise physiology to do this. Start with sports skills. If you want to be a good skier, volleyball player, or golfer, are your skills sufficient to achieve your goals? If you are like most people, you probably need work in this area. Have a coach or instructor help you develop a good skill-development program.

Next, assess your fitness. Are you strong or flexible enough to achieve your goals? A good way to assess your physical readiness for a sport is to compare yourself with successful people in your chosen activity (at the level you hope to achieve). To be a good recreational skier or tennis player, you should have the speed and stamina of people who play at that level. If you want to be a professional football player or Olympic shot-putter, you had better have the same strength and power as successful athletes, or you probably are not going to make it.

Do you have any injuries that have not healed? You can relieve chronic back, knee, and ankle pain with a systematic exercise program. Rather than making excuses, have a physician, physical therapist, or athletic trainer evaluate your injury, and start a rehabilitation program that will set you on the road to recovery.

Eat a Healthy Diet

The elements of a healthy, high-performance diet appear in Chapter 9. This diet is high in carbohydrates and low in fat, and it supplies enough calories, vitamins, and minerals to fulfill your body's nutritional needs. You do not need to buy expensive and unnecessary food supplements; you can eat a healthy, high-performance diet with foods available at the local supermarket. This diet will help you maintain a lean, healthy-looking body and will supply enough energy for your training program.

Train Your Mind

Consistent training is the key to developing fitness. This component takes discipline. Many people want instant results, but unfortunately, you get fit only after countless small steps. Gains are balanced with temporary setbacks and periods of stagnation. You have to develop the self-discipline to train consistently if you want to improve performance and fitness for sports and exercise.

Make training a priority. Develop enough mental discipline to go to the gym, swimming pool, or track regularly. Do not procrastinate; go to your workout on schedule. Often, people delay going to the gym. Consequently, they waste a lot of time. By the time they think about going to the workout, finally go to the gym, and "lollygag" around when they get there, they have spent two to three hours. Instead, they could have gone to the workout, finished it quickly, and returned home in about an hour. In short, develop the mental strength and discipline to exercise regularly.

Learn All You Can about Your Sport

A recurring theme of this book is that exercise training is as much art as it is science. The more you learn about the art and science of training and movement skills, the sooner you will develop a program that works for you.

Read as many books and magazine articles as you can about your favorite activities. Some of this information will be contradictory or poor quality. That is fine. With time, you will learn to extract useful information that will improve your training program.

Have Fun!

The following is an old saying among exercise critics: "Exercise doesn't make you live any longer; it just seems longer!" Your program does not have to be a chore if you choose activities you enjoy. If you do not like to jog, play tennis instead of running on a treadmill in the gym. If working out with friends motivates you, perhaps you should consider participating in aerobics classes at the local health club.

Masters-level competitive sports are extremely popular and are available for people ranging from college age to over 100 years. Training for track-and-field, volleyball, swimming, fun runs, cycling races and rallies, or softball adds purpose and enjoyment to your exercise program. You do not need to be an Olympic champion to participate in these sports. Every year, people in their fifties, sixties, and seventies take up these sports for the first time, and their only regret is that they did not take up these sports earlier. Masters sports are a great way to stay in shape, and they give purpose to your workouts.

Designing Your Program

First, determine your goals. If your goal is to improve your health, then your program will be quite simple. If you want to become a better skier, tennis player, golfer, body builder, or discus thrower, then your program becomes more complicated. To improve sports performance, you must balance skill and fitness development.

General Fitness for Health

Fitness for health was described in Chapter 3. To summarize, try to do a total of 30 minutes a day of some kind of exercise. The exercise does not have to be continuous; you could combine 15 minutes of walking to and from work with walking up stairs (instead of taking the elevator) and doing physically active household chores, such as mowing the lawn. Suggestions for becoming more physically active during the day are presented in Table 3.5. Ideally, you should supplement these exercises with resistance (Chapter 4) and flexibility exercises (Chapter 7). Make sure to combine your activity program with a well-balanced, low-fat diet (see Chapter 9).

Higher Levels of General Fitness

People interested in higher levels of general fitness should do some type of aerobic exercise 3–5 times per week (Chapter 3), resistance exercise 2–3 times per week, and flexibility exercises 5–7 times per week. If you want to become quicker and more powerful, include interval training and power and plyometric exercises in your program. This exercise program can be done at home, in a health club, or at the local track, park, or pool.

Choose aerobic exercises you enjoy. Possibilities include walking, running, swimming, aerobics classes, cross-country skiing, cycling, tennis, and basketball. Do aerobic exercise for at least 20 minutes. If you cannot do 20 minutes at first, build up to it gradually.

You can do resistance exercises on the same day as you do aerobic exercises. However, serious weight trainers often do resistance and aerobic exercises on

TABLE 8.2   Example of an Exercise Program to Develop Higher Levels of General Fitness

Components: Running, interval training, weight training, plyometrics, stretching, rest

Monday	Jog 2–3 miles in the park, stretching after your jog (5–10 exercises)
Tuesday	Weight training (3 sets of 10 repetitions): bench press, cleans, lat pulls or pull-ups, arm curls, crunches or sit-ups, squats or leg press, leg curls; stretching
Wednesday	Two miles interval training on track: stride or sprint the straightaways (100 meters), jog or walk the turns; plyometrics (3–6 exercises from Chapter 6); stretching
Thursday	Rest
Friday	Weight training (3 sets of 10 repetitions): squats or leg press, leg curls, cleans, bench press, lat pulls or pull-ups, arm curls, crunches or sit-ups; stretching
Saturday	Jog 2–3 miles in the park, stretching after your jog (5–10 exercises)
Sunday	Rest

separate days. For example, you might run on Monday, Wednesday, and Friday and lift weights on Tuesday and Thursday. Rest on Saturday and Sunday.

Do flexibility exercises at the end of your workouts because your muscles are warm and will stretch more than when they are cold. Also, you will be less susceptible to injury. Be consistent with your stretching. You can develop considerable flexibility by stretching for only 10 minutes a day. A sample exercise program to develop higher levels of general fitness is presented in Table 8.2.

Fitness Programs and Strength–Speed Sports

No single program exists that is appropriate for all sports. I will present two examples focusing on recreational (skier; see Table 8.3) and competitive athletes (football player; see Table 8.4) that will serve as templates. In general, during the off-season, develop your skills as well as your general strength, endurance, and flexibility fitness. As the season nears, place increasing emphasis on skill, power, and speed.

Your central goal is to develop movement skills in your sport. A tennis player who cannot serve or hit a good forehand or backhand will not play well in a match, no matter how good his or her physical fitness is. You will get the best results by systematically integrating fitness and skill.

SKILL DEVELOPMENT.   Both the competitive and recreational athlete should work on specific skills all year long. If your sport is seasonal, try to work on skills at least 2 days per week during the off-season. Make sure you practice the correct movements; repeating mistakes will only reinforce incorrect and poor movement patterns.

Do not use bad weather as an excuse. When it is raining, the tennis player can hit balls against a wall in the gym, the golfer can work on his or her swing at an

TABLE 8.3   Example of a Preseason Exercise Program to Develop Fitness for Alpine Skiing

Components: Skiing, running, interval training, weight training, plyometrics, stretching, rest

May–August: General fitness (see Table 8.2)

September–December

Monday	Weight training (3 sets of 10 repetitions): squats or leg press, leg curls, cleans, bench press, lat pulls or pull-ups, arm curls, crunches or sit-ups; jog 20–30 minutes on a treadmill; stretching
Tuesday	Two miles interval training on track: stride or sprint the straightaways (100 meters), jog or walk the turns; plyometrics (squat jumps, 360° squat jumps, ice skaters, standing long jumps, skiers, ski box jumps, long jumps); stretching
Wednesday	Weight training (3 sets of 10 repetitions): bench press, cleans, lat pulls or pull-ups, arm curls, crunches or sit-ups, squats or leg press, leg curls; stretching; jog 20–30 minutes on a treadmill, stretching after your jog (5–10 exercises)
Thursday	Rest
Friday	Weight training (3 sets of 10 repetitions): squats or leg press, leg curls, cleans, bench press, lat pulls or pull-ups, arm curls, crunches or sit-ups; jog 20–30 minutes on a treadmill; stretching
Saturday	Plyometrics, stadium stairs, cycling (bicycle or stationary bicycle) 40–60 minutes
Sunday	Rest

December–April

Monday	Rest
Tuesday	Two miles interval training on track: stride or sprint the straightaways (100 meters), jog or walk the turns; plyometrics (squat jumps, 360° squat jumps, ice skaters, standing long jumps, skiers, ski box jumps, long jumps); stretching
Wednesday	Weight training (3 sets of 10 repetitions): squats or leg press, leg curls, cleans, bench press, lat pulls or pull-ups, arm curls, crunches or sit-ups; jog 20–30 minutes on treadmill; stretching
Thursday	Two mile jog; plyometrics (squat jumps, 360° squat jumps, ice skaters, standing long jumps, skiers, ski box jumps, long jumps); stretching
Friday	Rest
Saturday–Sunday	Skiing

indoor range, and the discus thrower can work on turns in the garage. If all else fails, go to the local video store, and rent a movie about your favorite sport. Instructional films on skiing, golf, shot-putting, tennis, and softball are available.

During the season, increase the amount of time you practice your skills. During the golf, softball, tennis, or track seasons, practice skills at least 4 days per week. Do not substitute fitness for skill development. The golfer with a poor swing will shoot poorly, even if he or she can run fast or has a great bench press.

TABLE 8.4   Sample Exercise Program for Football

Football Season: Mid-August to November

December–April: 2 Week Cycles

Monday	Weight training: bench press (5 sets of 5 reps), cleans (5 × 5), support exercises (neck, arms, lats, abdomen, hamstrings, calves); jog 20–30 minutes on a treadmill or track; stretching
Tuesday	Football skills, 2 miles interval training on track: stride or sprint the straightaways (100 meters), jog or walk the turns; plyometrics (choose 6 exercises); stretching
Wednesday	Weight training: squats (5 × 5), snatch (5 × 3), support exercises; jog 20–30 minutes on a treadmill or track; stretching
Thursday	Rest
Friday	Weight training: bench press (5 sets of 5 reps), cleans (5 × 5), support exercises; jog 20–30 minutes on a treadmill or track; stretching
Saturday	Football skills, speed exercises, plyometrics, stadium stairs
Sunday	Rest
Monday	Weight training: squats (5 × 5), bench press (5 × 5), support exercises; jog 20–30 minutes on a treadmill or track; stretching
Tuesday	Football skills; speed exercises (e.g., 100 meter sprints, high knee exercise, harness sprints); plyometrics (choose 6 exercises); stretching
Wednesday	Weight training: cleans (5 × 3), jerks off the rack (5 × 3), support exercises; jog 20–30 minutes on a treadmill or track; stretching
Thursday	Rest
Friday	Weight training: squats (5 × 5), bench press (5 sets of 5 reps), support exercises; jog 20–30 minutes on a treadmill or track; stretching
Saturday	Football skills, speed exercises, plyometrics
Sunday	Rest

May–August: 2 Week Cycles

Monday	Football skills; weight training: bench press (5 sets of 2 reps), cleans (5 × 2), support exercises (neck, arms, lats, abdomen, hamstrings, calves); jog 20 minutes on a treadmill or track; stretching
Tuesday	Football skills; speed exercises (e.g., repeat 20–40 meter sprints, zigzag sprinting, high knee sprinting); plyometrics (choose 6 exercises); stretching
Wednesday	Weight training: squats (5 × 2), snatch (5 × 3), support exercises; jog 20 minutes on a treadmill or track; stretching
Thursday	Rest
Friday	Football skills; weight training: bench press (5 sets of 2 reps), cleans (5 × 2), support exercises; jog 20 minutes on a treadmill or track; stretching
Saturday	Football skills; speed exercises (e.g., repeat 20–40 meter sprints, zigzag sprinting, high knee sprinting); plyometrics (choose 6 exercises); stretching
Sunday	Rest

Monday	Football skills; weight training: squats (5 × 2), bench press (5 × 2), support exercises; jog 20 minutes on a treadmill or track; stretching
Tuesday	Football skills; speed exercises (e.g., 20–60 meter sprints, high knee exercises, harness sprints); plyometrics (choose 6 exercises); stretching
Wednesday	Weight training: cleans (5 × 3), jerks off the rack (5 × 3), support exercises; jog 20 minutes on a treadmill or track; stretching
Thursday	Rest
Friday	Football skills; weight training: squats (5 × 3), bench press (5 × 3), support exercises; jog 20–30 minutes on a treadmill or track; stretching
Saturday	Football skills; speed exercises (e.g., repeat 20–40 meter sprints, zigzag sprinting, backward sprinting, high knee sprinting); plyometrics (choose 6 exercises); stretching
Sunday	Rest

When combining sports and fitness, develop strength and endurance during the off-season, and as the season nears, place more emphasis on power, speed, and plyometric training. During the season, you still need to maintain your strength and endurance fitness.

BODYBUILDING.   Many people exercise so that they can build and maintain healthy, attractive-looking bodies. The basic principles behind a successful bodybuilding program are simple—build muscle tissue and minimize body fat. This principle is the same for men and women.

Bodybuilders generally complete a high number of sets and repetitions (5–10 sets of 10–15 repetitions) in a wide variety of exercises (10–25 exercises). Many successful bodybuilders also employ low-repetition, high-weight exercises for large-muscle groups, such as squats and bench presses.

Endurance training is important for bodybuilders. In addition to promoting health, it is an effective means of controlling body fat. Do your endurance exercise in the gym on a stair climbing machine, treadmill, or stationary bicycle; many people also enjoy outdoor activities, such as jogging in the park or cycling on the roads. A sample bodybuilding program is presented in Table 8.5.

ENDURANCE FITNESS.   Endurance sports are extremely popular throughout the world. Endurance races, such as the Bay-to-Breakers in San Francisco, the New York marathon, the Iron Man triathlon, and Western States 100, attract thousands of contestants, and lesser known races in running, cycling, swimming, triathlon, snow-shoeing, cross-country skiing, and rollerblading are held in almost every community of any size in the United States. Most contestants are not Olympic hopefuls. Rather, they are ordinary people who love endurance competitions and high levels of fitness. A sample program for a recreational distance runner is presented in Table 8.6.

TABLE 8.5   Sample Bodybuilding Program

Monday–Wednesday–Friday	Weight Training (use challenging weight for each set)
	  Bench press 5 × 10
	  Seated behind-the-neck press 4 × 10
	  Incline press 4 × 10
	  Lateral raises (dumbbells) 4 × 10
	  Front raises 4 × 10
	  Upright rowing 4 × 10
	  Pull-ups 3 × 10
	  Triceps extensions (lat machine) 3 × 10
	  Dumbbell curls 4 × 10
	  Triceps extensions on bench 3 × 10
	  Preacher curls 3 × 10
	  Squats 5 × 10
	  Sit-ups or crunches 5 × 25
	Aerobic exercise: 30–60 minutes (e.g., stairclimber, treadmill, stationary bicycle)
	Stretching (6–10 exercises)

Tuesday–Thursday	Aerobic exercise: 30 minutes Stretching
Saturday–Sunday	Rest

TABLE 8.6   Sample Program for Recreational Distance Runner

Monday	6 mile run Stretching
Tuesday	3 mile run Weight training: squats or leg presses (3 × 15), leg curls (3 × 15), sit-ups (3 × 25), bench presses (3 × 10), pull-ups (3 × 10), upright rowing (3 × 15) Stretching
Wednesday	Rest
Thursday	Interval training: 6–10 × 400 meters Stretching
Friday	3 mile run Weight training: squats or leg presses (3 × 15), leg curls (3 × 15), sit-ups (3 × 25), bench presses (3 × 10), pull-ups (3 × 10), upright rowing (3 × 15) Stretching
Saturday	6 mile run Stretching
Sunday	Rest

Endurance athletes should practice overdistance training to develop endurance capacity, interval training to develop speed and pace, and weight training to develop strength and power. During the off-season (time of year with few competitions), emphasize overdistance training. As the season nears, include more interval training workouts. Lift weights all year. During the competitive season, strive only to maintain strength by lifting weights 1–2 times per week.

Summary

As you can see, no one best training program for everyone is available. Rather, a loose set of training principles, if followed, will almost certainly lead to success. The most important thing is to keep exercising and have fun!

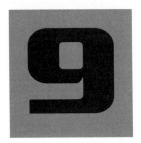

Nutrition for Health and Performance

Every day, you encounter a myriad of dietary information seeking to improve your eating habits. If you are not reading diet books that preach the latest weight-loss methods, you are carefully examining the nutritional contents of the foods you eat. Meanwhile, sports nutrition companies try to sell you their latest formula for improving performance. All this information is confusing. If you want to be an informed, health-conscious consumer, you need to know the principles of basic nutrition and weight control, not the latest diet crazes. Dietary information is important because good nutrition is critical for health, appearance, and performance.

Poor diet is linked to many degenerative diseases. To prevent coronary heart disease, some types of cancers, diabetes, and obesity, eat a proper diet. Dietary factors such as dietary fat, fiber, and vitamins greatly affect your health, longevity, and well-being.

Most people want to have a healthy, lean-looking body. However, you will probably never achieve this goal unless you pay attention to your diet. If you eat a lot of high-density, fatty foods, achieving the kind of body you want will be difficult—no matter how much you exercise. You must combine sensible eating and exercise habits to achieve the kind of body you want.

Sports and exercise performance depend on a good diet; the energy to run, jump, throw, and even rest comes from the foods you eat. Active people need a good diet to exercise and play sports effectively. Knowing what to eat and when can determine whether you run on empty during the day or have plenty of energy to work and play.

Many active people search for a magic nutritional formula to help them feel and perform better and control their weight. Consequently, they often take food supplements and drugs in the hope of reaching their goals. The performance nutrition industry is extremely competitive and markets a variety of products that promise to build muscle, enhance performance, and help people attain the perfect body. So, how do you separate reality from hype?

This chapter presents an overview of nutritional principles for health and performance. Topics include the elements of the healthy, high-performance diet, diet and weight control, and food supplements and performance-enhancing drugs.

Essential Nutrients

The six essential nutrients you need in your diet are fats, carbohydrates, proteins, vitamins, minerals, and water. Your body either does not produce these or makes them in insufficient quantities; therefore, you must include each component in your diet to stay alive and healthy.

You get energy from fats, carbohydrates, and proteins, while vitamins, minerals, and water help to regulate energy processes in your body. Nutrients drive your metabolism, which is all the chemical reactions occurring in your body. Running, jumping, throwing, skiing, and walking all require energy supplied by the food you eat. Proteins and fats are also used to make body structures, such as muscle, bone, and cell membranes.

Energy

Your ability to convert chemical energy from fuels to muscle energy (muscle contraction) mainly determines exercise performance. As you deplete your body's energy stores, you fatigue rapidly and performance decreases. Active people fight fatigue by including enough high-quality calories in their diet and restoring vital energy stores in muscles and the liver.

Fats provide the most energy, 9 kcal per gram; carbohydrates and proteins each supply 4 kcal per gram. Even alcohol, which is not an essential nutrient, supplies 7 kcal per gram. During the past fifteen years, experts have advised people to minimize the amount of fats they eat. High-fat diets, in addition to being extremely high in calories, also increase the risk of a variety of diseases.

The average adult needs about 2,000 kilocalories (kcal) per day, but if you are more active or larger than normal, you will need more calories. When you take in more calories than you use through metabolism or exercise, you will store the excess calories as fat.

Energy intake is important, even among people trying to lose weight. Starving yourself and overexercising can adversely affect your health, decrease performance, and make you feel miserable. When you try to lose weight, the best strategy is to decrease your caloric intake slightly and lose weight slowly. Weight-loss principles are discussed later in this chapter.

Most people take in more than enough kcal to supply their energy needs; in fact, overconsumption is a primary reason so many people are overweight. However, in extremely active people, underconsumption can be a problem. Nutritional studies of athletes show that the majority do not take in enough calories (Brooks et al., 2000). Calories are the most important nutritional factor for exercise performance;

inadequate caloric intake can lead to loss of body weight and muscle mass, depletion of carbohydrate stores in the muscles and liver, and sometimes low blood sugar during training.

Fats

Fats, also called lipids, are the most energy-rich food source and are mainly found in adipocytes (fat cells). You also store small amounts of fat in other cells, such as skeletal muscle. Even though many people try to carry as little fat as possible, it is far from being a useless tissue—it is the body's main energy-storage depot. It also protects and insulates your internal organs, comprises part of vital structures, such as cell membranes, and serves as a building block for many important hormones. Furthermore, dietary fats help you absorb some vitamins, serve as a vital energy source for most tissues in the body, help regulate several important body functions, such as blood pressure, and are critical for optimal fetal development during pregnancy.

Although several types of fats exist, the most important are triglycerides and cholesterol. Triglycerides are composed of glycerol and three fatty acids, which are classified according to their structure as saturated, monounsaturated, or polyunsaturated. Fats are saturated if they contain high amounts of saturated fatty acids. Foods with high saturated fat include meats, such as hamburger and steak, lunch meats, cheese, butter, and whole milk. Monounsaturated and polyunsaturated fats come from plants, such as olives, peanuts, corn, soybeans, and sunflowers. Although palm and coconut oil are from plant sources, they are highly saturated. Food manufacturers can also hydrogenate vegetable fats to make them saturated if they want to improve the texture of food and to increase the shelf life of their products.

Most people consume 30–40 percent of their calories as fat, yet the body needs only a fraction of this—about a tablespoon of vegetable oil a day. The high-fat diet increases serum cholesterol, a leading risk factor for coronary heart disease and some types of cancer. Nutritionists from the National Institute of Health recommend that fat intake be less than 30 percent of the calories you eat; some recommend even lower levels of fat intake (Brooks et al., 2000).

Restrict the amount of saturated fats in your diet. Better fat sources include olive oil, high in monounsaturated fatty acids, and most kinds of fish (e.g., salmon, trout, mackerel), which are high in omega-3 fatty acids. Omega-3 fatty acids are thought to reduce the risk of coronary heart disease (Nieman, 1999).

Consumer information on food containers makes it relatively easy to track your fat intake (Figure 9.1). The most important thing to look for on the label is the percentage of calories from fat. Try to eat foods in which fat constitutes 30 percent or less of the total calories, but you do not have to be fanatical. Fats add flavor to food. A hearty meal in a French restaurant would hardly be the same without some fats. Moderation is the key; if one food or meal contains more fat than is desirable, balance it with another food or a meal containing less than 30 percent fat. The important thing is to keep your fat content in your diet at 30 percent or less of your total calories.

Nutrition Facts

Serving Size   1 Box (43g)

Amount/serving	1 Box	Per 50g
Calories	160	180
Fat Calories	5	5

	% Daily Value**	
Total Fat 0.5g*	**1%**	**1%**
Saturated Fat 0g	**0%**	**0%**
Cholesterol 0mg	**0%**	**0%**
Sodium 270mg	**11%**	**13%**
Total Carb. 37g	**12%**	**14%**
Fiber 2g	**8%**	**8%**
Sugar 13g		
Other Carb. 22g		
Protein 3g		

	1 Box	Per 50g			1 Box	Per 50g
Vitamin A	10%	15%	•	Vitamin C	20%	25%
Calcium	0%	0%	•	Iron	80%	100%
Vitamin D	8%	10%	•	Vitamin E	80%	100%
Thiamin	80%	100%	•	Riboflavin	80%	100%
Niacin	80%	100%	•	Vitamin B$_6$	80%	100%
Folate	80%	100%	•	Vitamin B$_{12}$	80%	100%
Pantothenate	80%	100%	•	Phosphorus	8%	10%
Magnesium	6%	8%	• Zinc		80%	100%

* Percent Daily Values (DV) are based on a 2,000 calorie diet.

FIGURE 9.1   Sample Nutritional Information Label from Common Food Item.

Carbohydrates

Carbohydrates are the high-performance fuel—the most important energy source during exercise. The brain, nervous system, and blood cells depend on them as their fuel source. Your capacity for exercise and mental processing diminish quickly when you run out of this critical fuel.

Carbohydrates are classified as simple and complex. Simple carbohydrates contain only one to two sugar units per molecule; complex carbohydrates, on the other hand, consist of long chains of sugar molecules. Sweet-tasting foods such as table sugar and honey are examples of simple carbohydrates, and high-fiber foods such as fruits, some vegetables, and grains are complex carbohydrates. A diet high in dietary fiber is essential to maintain good gastrointestinal health and to prevent colon cancer. Nutritional experts recommend that you try to emphasize complex carbohydrates in your diet.

Your body controls blood sugar levels by absorbing carbohydrates from the food you eat and by breaking down stored carbohydrates. The latter process is particularly important when you need energy quickly, such as during exercise. Blood sugar is controlled by several important hormones—insulin, glucagon, and epinephrine (adrenaline); these hormones go to work when your body's energy level changes (e.g., after you have eaten a meal or during a workout). Although these hormones are critical to blood sugar regulation, they are ineffective unless they have fuels with which to work. Your body gets the carbohydrates it needs through the diet.

Carbohydrates are stored in cells as glycogen, which is a mass of blood sugar (glucose) units linked together. Your liver, kidneys, and muscles store most of your body's glycogen. During exercise, the most important carbohydrate source for muscular work is muscle glycogen; you use approximately six times more muscle glycogen than blood sugar to run, ride a bicycle, or lift weights. However, blood sugar is important because it fuels your nervous system. Without a well-functioning brain and nervous system, your motivation to train will stop, no matter how much glycogen you have stored in your muscles. Thus, you cannot neglect blood sugar when you consider which fuels your body will use during exercise. Although your muscle glycogen may provide most of the fuel for muscle movements, the blood glucose supplies the brains of the outfit.

Blood sugar can also be manufactured in the liver from amino acids, lactate (lactic acid without the acid), and pyruvate in a process called *gluconeogenesis.* Fuel sources flowing into the liver via the blood stream enter the liver, and it converts them into blood sugar. Through this process and by breaking down liver glycogen, your body can maintain reasonably high levels of blood sugar, even during prolonged fasting.

During exercise, blood sugar control processes allow blood sugar to increase. If you begin an exercise session with full glycogen stores in your liver, you can maintain elevated levels of blood sugar (compared to rest) for several hours of exercise before they begin to decline.

Unfortunately, the liver's storage capacity is limited. When you are on a prolonged, hard training program and do not eat enough calories or carbohydrates, liver glycogen stores can run low. Studies of athletes involved in heavy training show that because of poor diet, liver glycogen levels are often not optimal (Brooks et al., 2000). However, high-carbohydrate diets can maintain adequate glycogen stores in the liver. Eating a good breakfast is the best way to replenish liver stores after a long night without fuel intake.

Proteins

Proteins are the body's most important structural material, making up much of muscle, bone, enzymes, some hormones, and cell membranes, and are made of substances called amino acids. Of the twenty amino acids in foods, nine are considered essential in the diet because the body cannot make them. Essential amino acids include histidine, isoleucine, leucine, lysine, methionine, phenylalanine, theonine, tryptophan, and valine.

Protein supplements are popular with active people, particularly those who lift weights even though most people take in more protein than they need. The daily protein requirement is 0.8 grams of protein per kilogram body weight. People who are extremely active may need slightly more protein. However, since most U.S. athletes consume more than 1.5 grams of protein per kilogram body weight, a protein deficit in the diet is rarely a problem.

Proteins are important for people involved in endurance exercise because they help maintain blood sugar levels. The liver can convert amino acids to blood sugar through a process called gluconeogenesis, which literally means making new glucose or blood sugar. Gluconeogenesis helps the body maintain blood sugar during the hours between meals. Amino acids, the building blocks of proteins, break down slowly and act like time-released blood sugar tablets. Proteins in your meals help to maintain blood sugar for many hours and prevent hunger sensations.

Amino acid use, particularly of the branched-chain amino acids leucine, isoleucine, and valine, increases the longer and quicker you exercise. Protein in your meals can help restore depleted amino acids.

Vitamins and Minerals

In the United States, athletes and nonathletes spend incredible amounts of money on vitamin–mineral pills every year, yet the only commonly documented deficiency in the United States is iron deficiency. With a few possible exceptions, anything more than a balanced diet and a basic vitamin pill is useless and a waste of money.

Vitamins act as coenzymes (work with enzymes to drive the body's metabolism) and aid in the production and protection of red blood cells. Although vitamins are not produced in the body, they are required in extremely small amounts. Of all the body's vitamins, only vitamin C, thiamin, pyridoxine, and riboflavin are affected by exercise. Of these, only vitamin C supplementation has been shown to improve performance, and that was in only vitamin C-deficient adolescents (Nieman, 1999).

Vitamin C supplementation has been a fertile area of debate, since Linus Pauling suggested megadoses of the vitamin as a cure for the common cold. His contention has been extremely controversial, and, in general, medical studies have not supported his claims. However, recent studies have shown a link between vitamin C intake and immune function (Nieman, 1999). This link could be helpful to active people because preventing the downtime from illness can be as effective as discovering a new ergogenic aid to enhance performance. The debate regarding vitamin C and health will certainly continue for many years.

Vitamin supplements will improve performance only if there is a nutritional deficiency. Because a moderate increase in vitamin C intake is considered safe, it is not a bad idea to take basic vitamin supplements to compensate for an inadequate diet. Also, consuming additional vitamin C may be recommended in case it really does boost immune function. As long as excessive amounts of the vitamin are not consumed, the extra vitamin C probably will not harm you. However, there is no justification for the megadoses of vitamins taken by many athletes and active people.

Recent evidence suggests that vitamins C and E may also help to protect the body from destructive chemicals called free radicals, which your body produces naturally during metabolism. Cell damage from free radicals has been linked to aging and the breakdown of the immune function (Nieman, 1999). Vitamins C and E act as antioxidants that help eliminate free radicals and protect your body from their destructive effects. Scientists are now starting to learn about the relationship between vitamins and free radicals.

Water

Water makes up 60 percent of your body and is vitally important for controlling your metabolism, digesting food, delivering substances to your cells, enhancing cellular communication, and regulating temperature. Even a 2 percent drop in body water will affect your exercise performance.

Water is also found in almost all foods, particularly fruits, vegetables, and liquids. Although your body can produce water through metabolism, 80–90 percent of daily water turnover comes from your diet. Water intake must compensate for water losses. You lose water every day in urine, sweat, feces, and evaporation from the lung.

Water and salt intake affects your body water. Your body divides its water between cells, blood, and the area outside the cells. Dehydration upsets the balance, disrupts communications between different parts of the body, and results in poor coordination and muscle stiffness. You also lose salt from your body when you sweat. This loss can not only cause fluid problems but also induce muscle cramps.

The Healthy, High-Performance Diet and the Food Guide Pyramid

The basic principles of good nutrition include moderately eating a variety of foods in a balanced diet. It is difficult to improve on sensible eating habits for maximizing the effects of a fitness program and maintaining a trim, attractive body.

In 1995, the U.S. Department of Agriculture and the U.S. Department of Health and Human Services issued dietary guidelines for healthy U.S. citizens. The guidelines included a Food Guide Pyramid highlighting the elements of a well-balanced diet (Figure 9.2). A healthy diet plays a critical role in any fitness–nutrition program because it provides all of the known nutrients, reduces the risk of coronary artery disease and some types of cancer, and provides enough energy to sustain a vigorous training program. A balanced diet consists of at least three meals a day of foods chosen from six basic food groups:

- Bread, cereals, rice, and pasta: 6–12 servings
- Vegetables: 3–5 servings
- Fruits: 2–4 servings
- Meat, poultry, fish, dry beans, eggs, and nuts: 2–3 servings
- Milk, yogurt, and cheese: 2–3 servings
- Fats, oils, and sweets: No recommended servings

The food pyramid was designed to persuade people to eat fewer meat and dairy products containing cholesterol and saturated fats and to eat more cereals,

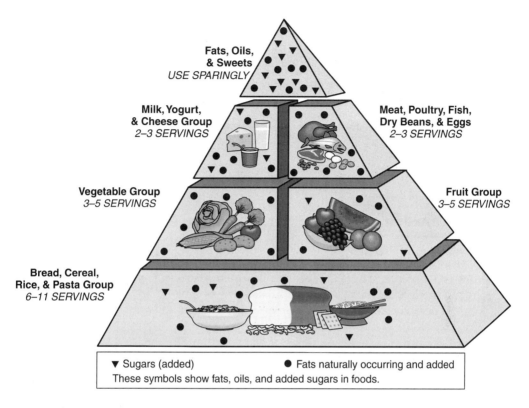

FIGURE 9.2   U.S. Department of Agriculture Food Guide Pyramid.

grains, fruits, and vegetables. The well-balanced diet suggested in the pyramid provides all known nutritional requirements and satisfies Recommended Daily Allowances (RDA) for important nutrients. Because all nutritional requirements possibly have not been identified, people should consume a variety of foods from the basic food groups. Remember, all the food supplements in the world are not going to make up for a poor diet. You cannot achieve optimal nutrition from a pill!

Milk and milk products are important sources of calcium, riboflavin, high-quality protein, carbohydrates, fat, and other assorted vitamins and minerals. Protein foods, such as meats, chicken, and fish, in addition to providing protein, also supply iron, thiamin, riboflavin, niacin, phosphorus, and zinc. Avoid eating meats with a high fat content because they are associated with increased risk of heart disease.

The cereals and grains, the lowest level of the pyramid, supply energy, thiamin, iron, niacin, and cellulose (fiber); these foods are critical for satisfying the energy requirements of a vigorous exercise program. Fruit and vegetables also supply vitamins, minerals, and fiber. You should eat dark green and deep yellow vegetables because of their high nutrient content and their possible influence in reducing the risk of certain types of cancer.

Diet, Exercise, and Weight Control

Your goal, which is not as easy as it sounds, when losing weight is to maintain muscle mass and lose fat. Most people want instant results. If your vacation or a class reunion is soon, you may try to lose weight in any way you can. Unfortunately, when you try to change your weight rapidly, the results are almost never satisfactory.

Rapid weight loss causes you to lose muscle. When you lose more than 3 pounds a week, 40–50 percent of the weight loss will be from lean body mass; your starving body uses your muscles for food. That is the last thing you need when you are trying to develop a fit, healthy-looking body.

Principles of Losing Weight for Active People

Weight loss is a worldwide obsession. Many people exercise hoping to keep their waistlines under control. However, a program that depends solely on exercise or diet is doomed to failure in the long run. You have to eat a healthy diet and exercise regularly if you want to achieve a fit, healthy-looking body.

The body's energy balance determines whether body fat increases, decreases, or remains the same. You gain fat when you eat more energy through meals than you burn through exercise and metabolism. Although exercise is an important part of a weight-control program, the successful program demands caloric restriction. Exercise alone is rarely effective. Fat loss occurs when you take in less food than the energy you use.

The goal of a weight-control program should be to lose body fat and maintain the loss. Quick-loss programs often result in the loss of muscle tissue and do nothing to instill healthy, long-term dietary habits that will maintain the new weight. Also, yo-yo diets are unhealthy, and they contribute to coronary heart disease. The following principles for losing body fat will increase the chances of success for your weight-control program.

STRESS FAT LOSS.   Rapid weight loss from fad diets usually causes loss of muscle mass and water; therefore, fat loss rather than weight loss should be the goal. Each pound of fat has 3,500 kcal. The energy requirement of the average active person (depending on size, gender, and activity level) is typically 2,000–5,000 kcal per day. Even if you ate nothing and your body used only fat for energy, you would lose body fat slowly.

LOSE WEIGHT SLOWLY.   Lose no more than 1 kg (2.2 lbs.) per week; more rapid weight loss results in the loss of muscle tissue. If you sustain a mild caloric deficit, you will lose fat and lose little muscle or water. The weight stays off better. When you lose muscle, your body's metabolism slows, and your need for food reduces. When you go back on your normal diet, you gain weight rapidly because you no longer need as much food as before.

EAT A BALANCED DIET.   Stress a balanced diet that is relatively high in complex carbohydrates and low in fat. Create a caloric deficit by combining caloric restriction with more exercise. Take in enough protein to help control appetite and maintain your muscles' needs. For active people, this is approximately 0.8–1 gram of protein per kilogram body weight a day. You will lose muscle if you cut your calorie intake by too much, regardless of how much protein you ingest.

EXERCISE REGULARLY.   Exercise is critically important for a successful weight-loss program. For the average person, the best exercises for losing weight include running, walking, and cycling. Exercise increases your metabolism both during and after the activity, which causes you to burn calories at a faster rate all day, and helps to maintain muscle mass, which is critical for maintaining metabolic rate. If you can maintain your muscle mass during weight loss, you will be more likely to maintain your new weight.

The best exercises for promoting fat loss are prolonged endurance exercises. However, doing intense exercise is also beneficial. High-intensity exercise increases your postexercise metabolism more than long–slow endurance exercise. Studies have also shown that you break down fats more quickly during the postexercise period after a high-intensity exercise workout (Brooks et al., 2000). High-intensity exercise also builds muscle mass more than slow-endurance training. The bottom line is that both prolonged endurance and high-intensity exercise are beneficial for weight control.

MONITOR BODY COMPOSITION.   Make sure that most weight loss is from a reduction in body fat rather than a reduction in lean-body mass. The best way to determine this is with an underwater weighing test, which is widely available in university exercise physiology laboratories, health clubs, and medical facilities. Every active person should know his or her body composition.

If you do not have access to underwater weighing, other methods are available. Perhaps the best is skin-fold calipers, available in almost every health club or high school physical education department. You can even buy plastic calipers from health-oriented magazines. Other popular methods include bioelectrical impedance and infrared methods. These techniques, while technologically advanced, are no more accurate than skinfolds.

AVOID WEIGHT LOSS AIDS.   The grocery and drugstore shelves are full of weight-loss products. Although research has shown that these over-the-counter drugs are mainly ineffective, several appetite-suppressing drugs, available by medical prescription, have been shown to be effective. However, almost all the patients gained back the weight they lost when they stopped taking the drugs. Also, the drugs had side effects, such as abnormal heart rhythms and insomnia (Brooks et al., 2000). The best advice is to stay away from drugs that promise to help you lose weight. They probably do not work, and if they do, they may damage your health.

The best strategy for body composition management is to lose weight (fat) slowly. Change your body composition gradually so that you gain muscle and lose fat. Rapid weight losses cause you to lose muscle and body water will impair your performance, and will not give you a healthy, fit-looking body.

Ergogenic Aids and Food Supplements

Substances taken to enhance performance are called *ergogenic aids*. Active people consume a variety of drugs and nutritional supplements in the quest for improved performance and the perfect body. They take these substances to (1) enhance muscle hypertrophy, (2) speed recovery and prevent the effects of overtraining, (3) increase training intensity and aggressiveness, and (4) control fat, body water, and appetite.

Fitness and bodybuilding have become popular, high-profile activities. Several bodybuilding champions have become international film stars, and many make a great deal of money endorsing athletic food supplements. Numerous bodybuilding and fitness magazines serve as promotional vehicles for many products of questionable value. As aware, educated fitness consumers, you should be able to separate fact from fiction when you evaluate performance-enhancing drugs and food supplements. This section of the chapter will review some of the more popular drugs and food supplements used by active people to promote appearance and performance.

Agents Taken to Promote Muscle Hypertrophy

This category concerns active people and constitutes the most significant area of abuse.

ANABOLIC–ANDROGENIC STEROIDS. People take anabolic steroids (AS) in the hope of gaining weight, muscle size, strength, power, speed, endurance, and aggressiveness. These drugs are widely used by both serious athletes and by active people trying to improve their appearance and performance.

In the United States in 1990, the Anabolic Steroid Control Act classified anabolic steroids as a Schedule III substance. The law gave the Drug Enforcement Administration (DEA) power to restrict the importation, exportation, distribution, and dispensation of anabolic steroids and has unfortunately led to a thriving black market for illegal anabolic steroids in the United States.

Anabolic steroids bind with receptor molecules in the cells and stimulate the cells to make proteins, an activity that enhances lean-body mass. They interfere with the activity of hormones that break down tissue after exercise, helping steroid users recover more quickly. Anabolic steroids may also increase aggressiveness, allowing athletes to train harder.

Side effects include liver toxicity and tumors, decreased high-density lipoproteins (good cholesterol), cardiac arrhythmia, reduced sperm count, lowered testosterone production, high blood pressure, increased risk of AIDS (because of shared needles), depressed immune function, glucose intolerance, psychological disturbances, masculinization in women and children, premature closure of the bone growth centers, and an increased cancer risk. Severe side effects of anabolic steroid use that have been reported in athletes, are myocardial infarction (heart attack), ventricular tachycardia (accelerated heart rate), liver cancer, and severe psychiatric disturbances. Athletes may be particularly prone to side effects because they often take high dosages of the drugs for prolonged periods of time.

GROWTH HORMONE. Growth hormone (GH) is popular with athletes because it increases muscle mass and strength. Reports in the news media suggest that, like anabolic steroids, its use has filtered down to nonathletic high school students (Brooks et al., 2000). The development of recombinant human growth hormone has made the hormone more widely available.

Growth hormone speeds the rate that proteins enter muscle cells, increasing their growth rate. It also stimulates another growth-promoting hormone called *insulin-like growth factor*. Growth hormone also mobilizes fats from the fat cells, so it is often used to help control body composition.

Human growth hormone studies have shown no beneficial effects on muscle or performance. Animal studies, on the other hand, found that growth hormone administration stimulates muscle growth. Observations in athletes suggest that GH is highly anabolic in intensely training elite bodybuilders; however, the side effects can be severe (Komi, 1992).

Prolonged growth hormone administration may result in low blood sugar, elevated insulin levels, insulin resistance, heart enlargement, and elevated blood fats. Long-term use could also lead to acromegaly, characterized by enlarged bones in the head, face, and hands, myopathy, peripheral nerve damage, weakening of the bones (osteoporosis), arthritis, and heart disease.

Some athletes also take drugs that increase natural growth hormone secretion. These drugs include propranolol, vasopressin, clonidine, and levodopa. Yet, there is no evidence that these practices enhance muscle hypertrophy.

INSULIN-LIKE GROWTH FACTOR (IGF-1). The use of recombinant IGF-1, also called somotomedin C, has recently become popular among athletes. Insulin-like growth hormone production is stimulated by growth hormone, and it is released mainly by the liver but may also be secreted by the testes, skeletal muscles, fat cells, bone, and heart. Insulin-like growth hormone is an extremely anabolic (muscle-building) hormone. The side effects are thought to be similar to those of growth hormone; long-term use may promote cancer growth.

DEHYDROEPIANDROSTERONE (DHEA) AND ANDROSTENEDIONE. Dehydroepiandrosterone and androstenedione are relatively weak androgen hormones that have effects similar to testosterone. They are widely available in health food stores and supermarkets. Athletes take this drug to stimulate muscle hypertrophy and to aid in weight control. Dehydroepiandrosterone and androstenedione administration in middle age and older adults resulted in improved energy levels, increased muscle mass, mental acuity, and immune function. However, these subjects had blood levels of the hormone at least 20 percent below the average level of a 20-year-old (Fahey, 1997). Their value as ergogenic aids may lie in their ability to increase serum testosterone concentrations.

High doses of DHEA (1,600 mg/d) in young men led to a reduction in HDL cholesterol (good cholesterol); however, in elderly subjects, DHEA reduced LDL (bad cholesterol) and had no effect on HDL. Doses of 150–300 mg/d have a marked effect on testosterone concentration, possibly leading to masculinization in women and interference with hormone controls in both sexes. Androstenedione administration could have similar side effects as DHEA.

INSULIN. Some active people take insulin injections to promote muscle hypertrophy. Insulin, aside from its influence on glucose and fat metabolism, affects protein metabolism. These effects include enhanced amino acid transport into cells, increased rate of incorporation of amino acids into protein, and suppression of protein breakdown. The effectiveness of insulin supplementation or elevation in stimulating muscle hypertrophy is not known. The most serious side effect of exogenous insulin administration in exercising bodybuilders is insulin shock, a condition where blood sugar reaches dangerously low levels.

CLENUBUTEROL. Athletes take this drug (a β2 adrenergic agonist) to prevent muscle atrophy, increase lean-body mass, and decrease body fat. Beneficial effects have been shown in animals, but few studies have been done in humans. Side effects include insomnia, abnormal heart rhythm, anxiety, depressed appetite, and nausea. More serious side effects include enlarged heart and heart attack.

OTHER AGENTS. Other agents sometimes used as ergogenic aids include human chorionic gonadotropin (HCG), periactin, conjugated linoleic acid (CLA), vanadyl sulfate, dibencozide, and organ extracts. These agents are less popular, and their effectiveness is questionable.

Agents Taken to Speed Recovery

The primary purposes of taking these agents are to replenish depleted body fuels (e.g., creatine phosphate: creatine supplementation; muscle and liver glycogen: glucose and lactate polymers) and to serve as a source for postexercise protein synthesis (e.g., amino acids).

CREATINE SUPPLEMENTATION. A recent survey suggests that currently, creatine (i.e., creatine monohydrate) is among the most popular and widely used supplements by athletes. They use these supplements to enhance recovery and exercise capacity.

Several studies have shown that creatine feeding (creatine monohydrate) increases the creatine phosphate content of the muscle by 20 percent by providing the muscles with an abundant source of creatine. The optimal dosage for achieving maximum values of muscle creatine is approximately 3–5 g/day (teaspoon); increasing the intake to 20 g/day resulted in no further increase in total muscle creatine. Creatine supplementation improved performance in short-term, high-intensity, repetitive exercise, which might make it a valuable supplement for active people (Fahey, 1997). It may improve performance by augmenting the availability of creatine phosphate and possibly regulating the rate of muscle sugar breakdown, and it may increase muscle building capacity during resistive exercise by allowing more intense training.

Creatine monohydrate supplementation has been associated with muscle cramping during and after exercise. Its long-term safety and effectiveness are currently unknown.

AMINO ACID AND POLYPEPTIDE SUPPLEMENTS. Athletes take amino acid and polypeptide supplements to accelerate muscle development, decrease body fat, and stimulate the release of growth hormone, yet there is little scientific proof to support amino acid or polypeptide supplementation. The protein requirement of active people is not much higher than sedentary individuals, so the rate of amino acid absorption from the gastrointestinal track is not important. Also, substituting amino acid or polypeptide supplements for protein-rich foods may cause deficiencies in important nutrients, such as iron and the B vitamins.

OTHER AGENTS. Carbohydrate beverages during and immediately following exercise enhance recovery from intense training, speeding up the replenishment of liver and muscle glycogen. The use of other substances to speed recovery, such as vitamin C, N-acetyl-L-Cysteine (NAC), inosine, and beta-hydroxy beta-methylbutyrate (HMB), is not currently supported by positive research findings (Costill & Miller, 1980).

Agents Taken to Increase Aggressiveness and Training Intensity

Serious exercisers often spend several hours per day training for their favorite activities. Monotony and fatigue sometimes deter significant improvement, so many athletes use stimulants to help them train harder and combat fatigue.

AMPHETAMINES. Some athletes and active people take amphetamines to prevent fatigue and to increase confidence and training intensity. Examples of amphetamines include benzedrine, dexedrine, dexamyl, and methedrine. These drugs stimulate the nervous system, causing increased blood pressure, increased heart rate, arousal, wakefulness, confidence, and the feeling of an enhanced capability to make decisions.

Studies show that the drugs mask fatigue but have not consistently shown that they increase endurance performance. Furthermore, most studies have shown increases in static strength but mixed results in muscle endurance. They appear to aid power-oriented movement skills in activities that employ constant motor patterns, such as shot putting and hammer throwing, and theoretically could provide some benefit to bodybuilders (Fahey, 1997).

However, amphetamines can also cause severe neural and psychological effects. These include aggressiveness, paranoia, hallucinations, compulsive behavior, restlessness, and irritability. In some cases, they can cause arrhythmias, hypertension, and angina (heart-related chest pain).

CAFFEINE.   Caffeine, found in coffee, cola, tea, and chocolate, is a favorite stimulant of active people. It stimulates the central nervous system by causing the release of adrenaline (epinephrine). In athletics, caffeine is used as a stimulant and as a fatty acid mobilizer. While there is some evidence that caffeine may improve endurance, the drug does not appear to enhance short-term, maximal exercise capacity (Fahey, 1997).

The diuretic and cardiac-stimulatory properties of this substance can combine to increase the risk of arrhythmias, such as ventricular ectopic beats and paroxysmal atrial tachycardia. Caffeine can also cause insomnia, and it is addictive.

OTHER AGENTS.   Other agents used by active people to enhance training intensity include cocaine, ephedrine, and ginseng. Cocaine use is not thought to be widespread in athletes, but some reportedly use it to increase training intensity. Ephedrine, a weak stimulant, is widely used by athletes during workouts; studies have shown that despite a slight stimulating effect on blood pressure and on exercise and recovery heart rates, ephedrine had no effect on physical work capacity (Fahey, 1997). Ginseng is also popular with athletes, but there is little evidence to support its use as an ergogenic aid.

Agents Taken to Aid Weight Control

Drugs used for weight control include those that suppress appetite, increase metabolic rate, affect the gastrointestinal tract, and control body water. Although some of these drugs may be temporarily effective, they can be dangerous and are not a satisfactory answer to long-term weight control.

The Polydrug and Food Supplement Phenomenon in Sports

The effects of the large variety and combination of supplements and drugs used by active people make it extremely difficult to determine the efficacy of these practices or precisely to predict the side effects. Numerous reports describe catastrophic side effects from unsafe drug use and nutritional supplementation. Learn all you can about these supplements before taking them. You will get the best results by following a sensible diet and training program and avoiding dubious and potentially dangerous drugs and supplements.

REFERENCES

Aagaard, P., and J. L. Andersen. 1998. Correlation between contractile strength and myosin heavy chain isoform composition in human skeletal muscle. *Med. Sci. Sports Exerc.* 30: 1217–1222.

ACSM position stand on the recommended quantity and quality of exercise for developing and maintaining cardiorespiratory and muscular fitness and flexibility in adults. 1998. *Med. Sci. Sports Exerc.* 30: 975–991.

Alter, M. J. 1988. *The Science of Stretching.* Champaign, IL: Human Kinetics.

American Association of Retired Persons (AARP). 1995. *Pep Up Your Life: A Fitness Book for Mid-Life and Older Persons.* Washington, D. C.: AARP, Fulfillment Department.

American College of Sports Medicine. 1992. *ACSM Fitness Book.* Champaign, IL: Human Kinetics.

American College of Sports Medicine. 1995. *ACSM's Guidelines for Exercise Testing and Prescription.* Baltimore: Williams and Wilkins (5th edition).

American Heart Association. 1995. *Exercise Standards: A Statement for Health Professionals.* Dallas, TX: American Heart Association.

American Medical Association, Council on Scientific Affairs. 1990. Medical and non-medical uses of anabolic-androgenic steroids. *JAMA* 264: 2923–2927.

Anderson, B. 1980. *Stretching.* Bolinas, CA: Shelter Publications.

Appleby, M., M. Fisher, and M. Martin. 1994. Myocardial infarction, hyperkalaemia and ventricular tachycardia in a young male body-builder. *Int. J. Cardiol.* 44: 171–174.

Armstrong, R. B., G. L. Warren, and J. A. Warren. 1991. Mechanisms of exercise-induced muscle fibre injury. *Sports Med.* 12: 184–207.

Atha, J. 1981. Strengthening muscle. *Exer. Sports Sci. Rev.* 9: 1–73.

Bahrke, M. S., C. E. Yesalosk, and J. E. Wright. 1990. Psychological and behavioral effects of endogenous testosterone levels and anabolic-androgenic steroids among males: A review. *Sports Med.* 10: 303–337.

Ballor, D. L., V. L. Katch, M. D. Becque, and C. R. Marks. 1988. Resistance weight training during caloric restriction enhances lean body weight maintenance. *Am. J. Clin. Nutr.* 47: 19–25.

Bandy, W. D., and J. M. Irion. 1994. The effect of time on static stretch on the flexibility of the hamstring muscles. *Phys. Ther.* 74: 845–852.

Beltz, S. D., and P. L. Doering. 1993. Efficacy of nutritional supplements used by athletes. *Clin. Pharm.* 12: 900–908.

Berg, A., I. Frey, M. W. Baumstark, M. Halle, and J. Keul. 1994. Physical activity and lipoprotein lipid disorders. *Sports Med.* 17: 6–21.

Berger, R. 1962. Optimum repetitions for the development of strength. *Res. Quart. Am. Alliance Health Phys. Educ. Recrea.* 33: 334–338.

Berger, R. 1963. Comparative effects of three weight training programs. *Res. Quart. Am. Alliance Health Phys. Educ. Recrea.* 34: 396–398.

Bergstrom, J., L. Hermansen, E. Hultman, and B. Saltin. 1967. Diet, muscle glycogen and physical performance. *Acta Physiol. Scand.* 71: 140–150.

Bijnen, F. C., C. J. Caspersen, and W. L. Mosterd. 1994. Physical inactivity as a risk factor for coronary heart disease: A WHO and International Society and Federation of Cardiology position statement. *Bull. World Health Organ.* 72 (1): 1–4.

Blackburn, J. R., and M. C. Morrissey. 1998. The relationship between open and closed kinetic chain strength of the lower limb and jumping performance. *J. Orthop. Sports Ther.* 27: 430–435.

Blair, S. N., H. W. Kohl, III, C. E. Barlow, R. S. Paffenbarger, Jr., L. W. Gibbons, and C. A. Macera. 1995. Changes in physical fitness and all-cause mortality. A prospective study of healthy and unhealthy men. *JAMA* 273 (14): 1093–1098.

Blamey, A., N. Mutrie, and T. Aitchison. 1995. Health promotion by encouraged use of stairs. *Br. Med. J.* 311: 289–290.

Bobbert, M. F. 1990. Drop jumping as a training method for jumping ability. *Sports Med.* 9: 7–22.

Bobbert, M. F., P. A. Huijing, and G. J. van Ingen Schenau. 1987. Drop jumping. I. The influence of jumping technique on the biomechanics of jumping. *Med. Sci. Sports Exerc.* 19: 332–338.

Brooks, G. A., and T. D. Fahey. 1987. *Fundamentals of Human Performance.* New York: Macmillan.

Brooks, G. A., T. D. Fahey, T. White, and K. Baldwin. 2000. *Exercise Physiology: Human Bioenergetics and Its Applications.* Mountain View, CA: Mayfield Publishing Co. (3rd edition).

Brown, C. H., and J. H. Wilmore. 1974. The effects of maximal resistance training on the strength and body composition of women athletes. *Med. Sci. Sport.* 6: 174–177.

Brown, R. D., and J. M. Harrison. 1986. The effects of a strength training program on the strength and self-concept of two female age groups. *Res. Quart. Sports Exerc.* 57: 315–320.

Buckley, W. E., C. E. Yasalis, K. E. Friedl, W. A. Anderson, A. L. Streit, and J. E. Wright. 1988. Estimated prevalence of anabolic steroid use among male high school seniors. *JAMA* 260: 3441–3445.

Butterfield, G., and D. Calloway. 1984. Physical activity improves protein utilization in young men. *Br. J. Nutr.* 51: 171–184.

Butts, N. K., K. M. Knox, and T. S. Foley. 1995. Energy costs of walking on a dual-action treadmill in men and women. *Med. Sci. Sports Exerc.* 27: 121–125.

Caiozzo, V. J., F. Haddad, M. J. Baker, and K. M. Baldwin. 1996. Influence of mechanical loading on myosin heavy-chain protein and mRNA isoform expression. *J. Appl. Physiol.* 80: 1503–1512.

Carmichael, C., and E. Burke. 1994. *Fitness Cycling.* Champaign, IL: Human Kinetics.

Carpinelli, R. N., and R. M. Otto. 1998. Strength training: Single versus multiple sets. *Sports Med.* 26: 73–84.

Castro, M. J., D. J. McCann, J. D. Shaffrath, and W. C. Adams. 1995. Peak torque per unit cross-sectional area differs between strength-trained and untrained young adults. *Med. Sci. Sports Exerc.* 27: 397–403.

Celejowa, I., and M. Homa. 1970. Food intake, nitrogen and energy balance in Polish weight lifters, during a training camp. *Nutr. and Met.* 12: 259–274.

Centers for Disease Control and Prevention. 1992. Prevalence of recommended levels of physical activity among women—Behavioral Risk Factor Surveillance System. *JAMA* 273 (13): 986–987.

Centers for Disease Control and Prevention. 1993. Public health focus: physical activity and the prevention of coronary heart disease. *JAMA* 270: 1529–1530.

Chilibeck, P. D., D. G. Sale, and C. E. Webber. 1995. Exercise and bone mineral density. *Sports Med.* 19: 103–122.

Chu, D. 1994. *Jumping into Plyometrics.* Champaign, IL: Leisure Press.

Clarkson, P. M., and D. J. Newham. 1997. Associations between muscle soreness, damage, and fatigue. *Adv. Exp. Med. Biol.* 384: 457–469.

Consolazio, C. F., H. L. Johnson, R. A. Dramise, and J. A. Skata. 1975. Protein metabolism during intensive physical training in the young adult. *Am. J. Clin. Nutr.* 28: 29–35.

Costill, D. L., E. F. Coyle, W. F. Fink, G. R. Lesmes, and F. A. Witzmann. 1979. Adaptations in skeletal muscle following strength training. *J. Appl. Physiol.* 46: 96–99.

Costill, D. L., and J. M. Miller. 1980. Nutrition for endurance sport: Carbohydrate and fluid balance. *Int. J. Sports Med.* 1: 2–14.

Coyle, E. F. 1995. Substrate utilization during exercise in active people. *Am. J. Clin. Nutr.* 61 (4 Suppl): 968S–979S.

Coyle, E. F., S. Bell, D. L. Costill, and W. J. Fink. 1978. Skeletal muscle fiber characteristics of world class shot-putters. *Res. Quart.* 49: 278–284.

Darden, E. 1982. *The Nautilus Bodybuilding Book.* Chicago: Contemporary Books.

Darden, E. 1984. *The Nautilus Advanced Bodybuilding Book.* New York: Simon & Schuster.

Delecluse, C. 1997. Influence of strength training on sprint running performance. *Sports Med.* 24: 147–156.

DeLorme, R., and F. Stransky. 1990. *Fitness and Fallacies.* Dubuque, IA: Kendall/Hunt.

Department of Health and Human Services. 1996. *Physical Activity and Health: A Report of the Surgeon General.* Atlanta: U.S. Department of Health and Human Services, Centers for Disease Control and Prevention, National Center for Chronic Disease Prevention and Health Promotion.

Despres, J. P., and B. Lamarche. 1994. Low-intensity endurance exercise training, plasma lipoproteins, and the risk of coronary heart disease. *J. Intern. Med.* 236: 7–22.

Dishman, R. K. 1994. Prescribing exercise intensity for healthy adults using perceived exertion. *Med. Sci. Sports Exerc.* 26: 1087–1094.

Dons, B., K. Bollerup, F. Bonde-Petersen, and S. Hancke. 1979. The effect of weight-lifting exercise related to muscle fiber composition and muscle cross-sectional area in humans. *Eur. J. Appl. Physiol.* 40: 95–106.

Edgerton, V. R. 1976. Neuromuscular adaptation to power and endurance work. *Can. J. Appl. Sports Sci.* 1: 49–58.

Edgerton, V. R. 1978. Mammalian muscle fiber types and their adaptability. *Amer. Zool.* 18: 113–125.

Enoka, R. M. 1988. Muscle strength and its development. *Sports Med.* 6: 146–168.

Fahey, T. D. 1987. *Athletic Training: Principles and Practice.* Mountain View, CA: Mayfield Publishing Co.

Fahey, T. 1997. Pharmacology of bodybuilding. In *The Clinical Pharmacology of Sport and Exercise.* Amsterdam: Elsevier Science B.V.

Fahey, T. D. 2000. *Basic Weight Training for Men and Women.* Mountain View, CA: Mayfield Publishing Co. (4th edition).

Fahey, T. D., L. Akka, and R. Rolph. 1975. Body composition and $\dot{V}O_{2max}$ of exceptional weight-trained athletes. *J. Appl. Physiol.* 39: 559–561.

Fahey, T. D., and G. Hutchinson. 1992. *Weight Training for Women.* Mountain View, CA: Mayfield Publishing Co.

Fahey, T. D., P. M. Insel, and W. T. Roth. 1999. *Fit and Well.* Mountain View, CA: Mayfield Publishing Co. (3rd edition).

Fahey, T. D., and M. S. Pearl. 1998. The hormonal and perceptive effects of phosphatidylserine administration during two weeks of resistive exercise-induced overtraining. *Biol. Sport.* 15: 135–144.

Fleck, S. J., and W. J. Kraemer. 1997. *Designing Resistance Training Programs.* Champaign, IL: Human Kinetics.

Florini, J. R. 1987. Hormonal control of muscle growth. *Mus. Ner.* 10: 577–598.

Fnes, J. E. 1994. *Living Well.* Reading, MA: Addison-Wesley.

Fowler, N. E., Z. Trzaskoma, A. Wit, L. Iskra, and A. Lees. 1995. The effectiveness of a pendulum swing for the development of leg strength and counter-movement jump performance. *J. Sports Sci.* 13: 101–108.

Friedlander, A. L., H. K. Genant, S. Sadowsky, N. N. Byl, and C. C. Gluer. 1995. A two-year program of aerobics and weight training enhances bone mineral density of young women. *J. Bone Miner. Res.* 10: 574–585.

Garfinkle, S., and E. Cafarelli. 1992. Relative changes in maximal force, EMG, and muscle cross-sectional area after isometric training. *Med. Sci. Sports Exerc.* 24: 1220–1227.

Garhammer, J. 1980. Power production by Olympic weightlifters. *Med. Sci. Sports Exerc.* 12: 54–60.

Garhammer, J. 1991. A comparison of maximal power outputs between elite male and female weightlifters in competition. *Int. J. Sports Biomech.* 7: 3–11.

Gillette, C. A., R. C. Bullough, and C. L. Melby. Postexercise energy expenditure in response to acute aerobic or resistive exercise. 1994. *Int. J. Sports Nutr.* 4: 347–360.

Goldberg, A. L. 1972. Mechanisms of growth and atrophy of skeletal muscle. In R. G. Cassens, (Ed.), *Muscle Biology.* New York: Marcel Dekker, Inc.

Gollnick, P. D., R. B. Armstrong, C. W. Saubertt, K. Piehl, and B. Saltin. 1972. Enzyme activity and fiber composition in skeletal muscle of trained and untrained men. *J. Appl. Physiol.* 33: 312–319.

Gonyea, W. J., and D. Sale. 1982. Physiology of weight lifting. *Arch. Phys. Med. Rehabil.* 63: 235–237.

Greendale, G. A., E. Barrett-Connor, S. Edelstein, S. Ingles, and R. Haile. 1995. Lifetime leisure exercise and osteoporosis. The Rancho Bernardo study. *Am. J. Epidemiol.* 141: 951–959.

Hakkinen, K., A. Pakarinen, and M. Kallinen. 1992. Neuromuscular adaptations and serum hormones in women during short-term intensive strength training. *Eur. J. Appl. Physiol.* 64: 106–111.

Harridge, S. D., R. Bottinelli, M. Canepari, M. Pellegrino, C. Reggiani, M. Esbjornsson, P. D. Balsom, and B. Saltin. 1998. Sprint training, *in vitro* and *in vivo* muscle function, and myosin heavy chain expression. *J. Appl. Physiol.* 84: 442–449.

Haskell, W. L. J. B. Wolffe Memorial Lecture. 1994. Health consequences of physical activity: Understanding and challenges regarding dose-response. *Med. Sci. Sports Exerc.* 26 (6): 649–660.

Haskell, W. L., J. Scala, and J. Whittam, eds. 1982. *Nutrition and Athletic Performance.* Palo Alto, CA: Bull Publishing.

Heath, G. W., and J. D. Smith. 1994. Physical activity patterns among adults in Georgia: Results from the 1990 Behavioral Risk Factor Surveillance System. *South. Med. J.* 87 (4): 435–439.

Heyward, V. H. 1991. *Advanced Fitness Assessment & Exercise Prescription.* Champaign, IL: Human Kinetics (2nd edition).

Hickson, R. C. 1980. Interference of strength development by simultaneously training for strength and endurance. *Eur. J. Appl. Physiol.* 45: 255–263.

Higbie, E. J., K. J. Cureton, G. L. Warren, III, and B. M. Prior. 1996. Effects of concentric and eccentric training on muscle strength, cross-sectional area, and neural activation. *J. Appl. Physiol.* 81: 2173–2181.

Hill, A. V. 1970. *First and Last Experiments in Muscle Mechanics.* Cambridge: Cambridge University Press.

Hortobagyi, T., J. P. Hill, J. A. Houmard, D. D. Fraser, N. J. Lambert, and R. G. Israel. 1996. Adaptive responses to muscle lengthening and shortening in humans. *J. Appl. Physiol.* 80: 765–772.

Huey, L., and R. Forster. 1993. *The Complete Waterpower Workout Book.* New York: Random House.

Huie, M. J. 1994. An acute myocardial infarction occurring in an anabolic steroid user. *Med. Sci. Sports Exerc.* 26: 408–413.

Israel, R. G., M. J. Sullivan, R. H. Marks, R. S. Cayton, and T. C. Chenier. 1994. Relationship between cardiorespiratory fitness and lipoprotein(a) in men and women. *Med. Sci. Sports Exerc.* 26: 425–431.

Johnson, R., and B. Tulin. 1995. *Travel Fitness.* Champaign, IL: Human Kinetics.

Jones, T. F., and C. B. Eaton. 1995. Exercise prescription. *Am. Fam. Physician* 52: 543–550, 553–555.

Kawakami, Y., T. Abe, and T. Fukunaga. 1993. Muscle-fiber pennation angles are greater in hypertrophied than in normal muscles. *J. Appl. Physiol.* 74: 2740–2744.

Kelley, G. 1996. Mechanical overload and skeletal muscle fiber hyperplasia: A meta-analysis. *J Appl. Physiol.* 81: 1584–1588.

King, A. C., W. L. Haskell, D. R. Young, R. K. Oka, and M. L. Stefanick. 1995. Long-term effects of varying intensities and formats of physical activity on participation rates, fitness, and lipoproteins in men and women aged 50 to 65 years. *Circulation* 91 (10): 2596–2604.

King, A. C., and D. L. Tribble. 1991. The role of exercise in weight regulation in nonathletes. *Sports Med.* 11: 331–349.

Kleiber, M. 1961. *The Fire of Life.* New York: Wiley & Sons.

Kline, G. M., J. P. Porcari, R. Hintermeister, P. S. Freedson, A. Ward, R. F. McCarron, J. Ross, and J. M. Rippe. 1987. Estimation of $\dot{V}O_{2max}$ from a one-mile track walk, gender, age, and body weight. *Med. Sci. Sports Exerc.* 19: 253–259.

Knapik, J. J., B. H. Jones, C. L. Bauman, and J. M. Harris. 1992. Strength, flexibility and athletic injuries. *Sports Med.* 14: 277–288.

Komi, P. V. 1984. Physiological and biomechanical correlates of muscle function: Effects of muscle structure and stretch-shortening cycle on force and speed. *Exer. Sci. Sports Rev.* 12: 81–121.

Komi, P. V. 1986. Training of muscle strength and power: Interaction of neuromotoric, hypertrophic, and mechanical factors. *Int. J. Sports Med.* 7: 10–15.

Komi, P. V., ed. 1992. *Strength and Power in Sport.* London: Blackwell Scientific Publications.

Kraemer, W. J. 1988. Endocrine responses to resistance exercise. *Med. Sci. Sports Exerc.* 20 (Suppl.): S152–157.

Kraemer, W. J., J. F. Patton, S. E. Gordon, E. A. Harman, M. R. Deschenes, K. Reynolds, R. U. Newton, N. T. Triplett, and J. E. Dziados. 1995.

Compatibility of high-intensity strength and endurance training on hormonal and skeletal muscle adaptations. *J. Appl. Physiol.* 78: 976–989.

Kuramoto, A. K., and V. G. Payne. 1995. Predicting muscular strength in women: A preliminary study. *Res. Q. Exerc. Sport* 66: 168–172.

Lemon, P. W. R. 1987. Protein and exercise. *Med. Sci. Sports Exerc.* 19 (Suppl.): 179–190.

Lesmes, G. R., D. Costill, E. F. Coyle, and W. J. Fink. 1978. Muscle strength and power changes during maximal isokinetic training. *Med. Sci. Sports* 10: 266–269.

Leterme, D., C. Cordonnier, Y. Mounier, and M. Falempin. 1994. Influence of chronic stretching upon rat soleus muscle during non-weight-bearing conditions. *Pflugers Arch.* 429: 274–279.

Linderman, J., T. D. Fahey, L. Kirk, J. Musselman, and B. Dolinar. 1992. The effects of sodium bicarbonate and pyridoxine-alpha-ketoglutarate on short-term maximal exercise capacity. *J. Sports Sci.* 10: 243–253.

Lombard, D. N., T. N. Lombard, and R. A. Winett. 1995. Walking to meet health guidelines: The effect of prompting frequency and prompt structure. *Health Psychol.* 14: 164–170.

Lycholat, T. 1995. *The Complete Book of Stretching.* Wiltshire, England: Crowood (2nd ed.).

McCall, G. E., W. C. Byrnes, A. Dickinson, P. M. Pattany, and S. J. Fleck. 1996. Muscle fiber hypertrophy, hyperplasia, and capillary density in college men after resistance training. *J. Appl. Physiol.* 81: 2004–2012.

McCarthy, J. P., J. C. Agre, B. K. Graf, M. A. Pozniak, and A. C. Vailas. 1995. Compatibility of adaptive responses with combining strength and endurance training. *Med. Sci. Sports Exerc.* 27: 429–436.

MacDougall, J. D. 1992. *Physiological Testing of the High-Performance Athlete.* Champaign, IL: Human Kinetics (2nd edition).

MacIntyre, D. L., W. D. Reid, and D. C. McKenzie. 1995. Delayed muscle soreness. The inflammatory response to muscle injury and its clinical implications. *Sports Med.* 20: 24–40.

Mastropaolo, J. A. 1992. A test of the maximum-power theory for strength. *Eur. J. Appl. Physiol.* 65: 415–420.

Melpomene Institute for Women's Health Research. 1990. *The Bodywise Woman.* Champaign, IL: Human Kinetics.

Mills, E. M. 1994. The effect of low-intensity aerobic exercise on muscle strength, flexibility, and balance among sedentary elderly persons. *Nurs. Res.* 43: 207–211.

Moritani, T., and H. A. deVries. 1979. Neural factors versus hypertrophy in the time course of muscle strength gain. *Amer. J. Phys. Med.* 58: 115–130.

Nardone, A., C. Romanò, and M. Schieppatgi. 1989. Selective recruitment of high-threshold human motor units during voluntary isotonic lengthening of active muscles. *J. Physiol.* 409: 451–471.

National Strength and Conditioning Association. 1989. Strength training for female athletes: A position paper. Part I. *Nat. Strength Condit. Assoc. J.* 11: 43–56.

Nieman, D. C. 1995. *Fitness and Sports Medicine: A Health Related Approach.* Palo Alto, CA: Bull Publishing.

Nieman, D. C. 1999. *Exercise Testing and Prescription.* Mountain View, CA: Mayfield Publishing Co.

O'Shea, P. 1964. Effects of selected weight training programs on the development of strength and muscle hypertrophy. *Res. Quart.* 37: 95–102.

Osternig, L. R., R. H. Robertson, R. K. Troxel, and P. Hansen. 1990. Differential responses to proprioceptive neuromuscular facilitation (PNF) stretch techniques. *Med. Sci. Sports Exerc.* 22: 106–111.

Pate, R. R., M. Pratt, S. N. Blair, W. L. Haskell, C. A. Macera, C. Bouchard, D. Buchner, W. Ettinger, G. W. Heath, and A. C. King, et al. 1995. Physical activity and public health. A recommendation from the Centers for Disease Control and Prevention and the American College of Sports Medicine. *JAMA* 273 (5): 402–407.

Peterson, G. E., and T. D. Fahey. 1984. HDL-C in five elite athletes using anabolic-androgenic steroids. *Physician Sportsmed.* 12 (6): 120–130.

Pierce, E. F., S. W. Butterworth, T. D. Lynn, J. O'Shea, and W. G. Hammer. 1992. Fitness profiles and activity patterns of entering college students. *J. Am. Coll. Health* 41: 59–62.

Rodriguez, B. L., J. D. Curb, C. M. Burchfield, R. D. Abbott, H. Petrovitch, K. Masaki, and D. Chiu. 1994. Physical activity and 23-year incidence of coronary heart disease morbidity and mortality among middle-aged men. The Honolulu Heart Program. *Circulation* 89: 2540–2544.

Rogozkin, V. 1988. *Metabolism of Anabolic Androgenic Steroids.* St. Petersburg, Russia: Hayka.

Rooney, K. J., R. D. Herbert, and R. J. Balnave. 1994. Fatigue contributes to the strength training stimulus. *Med. Sci. Sports Exerc.* 26: 1160–1164.

Rosenberg, I. H. 1994. Keys to a longer, healthier, more vital life. *Nutr. Rev.* 52 (8, Pt. 2): S50–51.

Sale, D. G. 1988. Neural adaptation to resistance training. *Med. Sci. Sports Exerc.* 20 (Suppl.): S135-S145.

Sale, J. E., L. J. McCargar, S. M. Crawford, and J. E. Taunton. 1995. Effects of exercise modality on metabolic rate and body composition. *Clin. J. Sports Med.* 5: 100–107.

Saltin, B., and P. D. Gollnick. 1983. Skeletal muscle adaptability: Significance for metabolism and performance. In *Handbook of Physiology. Skeletal Muscle* (pp. 555–631). Bethesda, MD: Am. Physiol. Soc.

Schroeder, R. 1990. *Assessing Fitness.* Dubuque, IA: Kendall Hunt.

Shangold, M., and G. Merkin. (Eds.). 1994. *Women and Exercise: Physiology and Sports Medicine.* Philadelphia: F. A. Davis (2nd edition).

Shephard, R. J. 1994. *Aerobic Fitness and Health.* Champaign, IL: Human Kinetics.

Shephard, R. J., T. Kavanagh, D. J. Mertens, S. Qureshi, and M. Clark. 1995. Personal health benefits of Masters athletics competition. *Br. J. Sports Med.* 29: 35–40.

Shephard, R. J., and P. N. Shek. 1995. Cancer, immune function, and physical activity. *Can. J. Appl. Physiol.* 20: 1–25.

Siegel, P. Z., R. M. Brackbill, and G. W. Heath. 1995. The epidemiology of walking for exercise: Implications for promoting activity among sedentary groups. *Am. J. Public Health* 85 (5): 706–710.

Silvester, L. J., C. Stiggins, C. McGown, and G. R. Bryce. 1982. The effects of variable resistance and free-weight training on strength and vertical jump. *Nat. Strength Cond. Assoc. J.* 3: 30–33.

Simoes, E. J., T. Byers, R. J. Coates, M. K. Serdula, A. H. Mokdad, and G. W. Heath. 1995. The association between leisure-time physical activity and dietary fat in American adults. *Am. J. Public Health* 85 (2): 240–244.

Smith, C. A. 1994. The warm-up procedure: To stretch or not to stretch. A brief review. *J. Orthop. Sports Phys. Ther.* 19: 12–17.

Sobel, D., and A. C. Klein. 1994. *Backache: What Exercises Work.* New York: St. Martin's.

Soest, A. J. van, and M. F. Bobbert. 1993. The role of muscle properties in control of explosive movements. *Biol. Cybern.* 69: 195–204.

Staron, R. S., F. C. Hagerman, and R. S. Hikida. 1981. The effects of detraining on an elite power lifter. *J. Neur. Sci.* 51: 247–257.

Stutz, David R., and the editors of Consumer Reports Books. 1994. *40+ Guide to Fitness.* Yonkers, NY: Consumers Union of the United States, Inc.

Tesch, P. A., and L. Larsson. 1982. Muscle hypertrophy in bodybuilders. *Eur. J. Appl. Physiol.* 49: 301–306.

Thomis, M. A. I., G. P. Beunen, H. H. Maes, C. J. Blimkie, M. Van Leemputte, A. L. Claessens, G. Marchal, E. Willems, and R. F. Vlietinck. 1998. Strength training: Importance of genetic factors. *Med. Sci. Sports Exerc.* 30: 724–731.

Thorstensson, A. 1976. Muscle strength, fibre types and enzyme activities in man. *Acta Physiol. Scand.* 443 (Suppl.): 1–45.

Tobias, M., and J. Sullivan. 1994. *Complete Stretching.* New York: Knopf.

Treuth, M. S., G. R. Hunter, T. Kekes-Szabo, R. L. Weinsier, M. I. Goran, and L. Berland. 1995. Reduction in intra-abdominal adipose tissue after strength training in older women. *J. Appl. Physiol.* 78: 1425–1431.

Viru, A., and T. Smirnova. 1995. Health promotion and exercise training. *Sports Med.* 19: 123–136.

Walberg, J. L. 1989. Aerobic exercise and resistance weight-training during weight reduction. *Sports Med.* 47: 343–356.

Welle, S., C. Thornton, and M. Statt. 1995. Myofibrillar protein synthesis in young and old human subjects after three months of resistance training. *Am. J. Physiol.* 268: E422–427.

Wells, C. L. 1985. *Women. Sport and Performance.* Champaign, IL: Human Kinetics.

Williams, M. H. (Ed.). 1983. *Ergogenic Aids in Sport.* Champaign, IL: Human Kinetics.

Williams, M. H. 1994. The use of nutritional ergogenic aids in sports: Is it an ethical issue? *Int. J. Sports Nutr.* 4: 120–131.

Williams, P. E., T. Cantanese, E. G. Lucey, and G. Goldspink. 1988. The importance of stretch and contractile activity in the prevention of connective tissue accumulation in muscle. *J. Anat.* 158: 109–114.

Wilson, G. J., A. J. Murphy, and A. Walshe. 1996. The specificity of strength training: The effect of posture. *Eur. J. Appl. Physiol.* 73: 346–352.

Worrell, T. W., T. L. Smith, and J. Winegardner. 1994. Effect of hamstring stretching on hamstring muscle performance. *J. Orthop. Sports Phys. Ther.* 20: 154–159.

Wright, J. 1980. Anabolic steroids and athletics. *Exer. Sports Sci. Rev.* 8: 149–202.

YMCA, and T. W. Hanlon. 1995. *Fit for Two: The Official YMCA Prenatal Exercise Guide.* Champaign, IL: Human Kinetics.

INDEX